The Client's Guide to Therapy

How to Get the Most out of Your Counseling Experience

Terri S. Watson, PsyD

ivp
Academic
An imprint of InterVarsity Press
Downers Grove, Illinois

InterVarsity Press
P.O. Box 1400 | Downers Grove, IL 60515-1426
ivpress.com | email@ivpress.com

©2025 by Terri S. Watson

InterVarsity Press® is the publishing division of InterVarsity Christian Fellowship/USA®. For more information, visit intervarsity.org.

All Scripture quotations, unless otherwise indicated, are taken from The Holy Bible, New International Version®, NIV®. Copyright © 1973, 1978, 1984, 2011 by Biblica, Inc.™ Used by permission of Zondervan. All rights reserved worldwide. www.zondervan.com. The "NIV" and "New International Version" are trademarks registered in the United States Patent and Trademark Office by Biblica, Inc.™

While any stories in this book are true, some names and identifying information may have been changed to protect the privacy of individuals.

The publisher cannot verify the accuracy or functionality of website URLs used in this book beyond the date of publication.

Cover design: Faceout Studios
Interior design: Jeanna Wiggins

ISBN 978-1-5140-0882-9 (print) | ISBN 978-1-5140-0883-6 (digital)

Printed in the United States of America ∞

Library of Congress Cataloging-in-Publication Data
Names: Watson, Terri S., 1959- author.
Title: The client's guide to therapy : how to get the most out of your
   counseling experience / Terri S. Watson.
Description: Downers Grove, IL : IVP Academic, [2025] | Includes
   bibliographical references and index.
Identifiers: LCCN 2024040518 (print) | LCCN 2024040519 (ebook) | ISBN
   9781514008829 (print) | ISBN 9781514008836 (digital)
Subjects: LCSH: Psychotherapy–Religious aspects–Christianity. |
   Psychotherapy–Popular works.
Classification: LCC RC489.S676 W38 2025 (print) | LCC RC489.S676 (ebook)
   | DDC 616.89/14–dc23/eng/20241207
LC record available at https://lccn.loc.gov/2024040518
LC ebook record available at https://lccn.loc.gov/2024040519

32   31   30   29   28   27   26   25 | 13   12   11   10   9   8   7   6   5   4   3   2   1

To my beloved clients:

I dedicate this book with gratitude

for the sacred calling to be part of your

courageous and inspiring journeys

over these many years.

Important Note

If you or someone you know is currently experiencing active thoughts of harming yourself or someone else, or is having a mental health crisis, please call 911 or go to your local emergency room. You can also call or text the Suicide and Crisis Line at 988 to speak confidentially with a crisis counselor. For international assistance, Find a Helpline is an excellent online resource to identify crisis support by country at **www.iasp.info/crisis-centres-helplines**.

Contents

Acknowledgments

This book reflects the formative influences of many important people who have shaped my understanding of the art and science of psychotherapy. I am grateful to God for their influence on my life and work.

To my clients—past, present, and future—you have my deepest appreciation for all you have taught me about growth, transformation, and spiritual fortitude. You will always have my enduring love and appreciation for the therapist I am today.

To the faculty, staff, and students in the School of Psychology, Counseling and Family Therapy at Wheaton College—thank you for instilling in me a vision for therapy as ministry to the marginalized and the global church. It has been truly an honor to be part of this remarkable educational community throughout my whole adult life in many different roles—graduate student, new faculty member, program director, dean, and tenured professor. To the Wheaton alumni serving around the world (you know who you are!)—you inspire me every day!

To my therapist colleagues who have modeled and inspired a view of our work as a holy calling, thank you. Our conversations over the years have been essential and impactful, as you will see reflected in the following pages. I am especially grateful to the organizations that sponsor annual conferences for therapists to engage in important conversations about faith integration in counseling and psychology, including the Christian Association for Psychological Studies conference and the Mental Health and Missions conference (sponsored by Mission Training International).

A special thanks to those who have been essential to the development of this book project, especially InterVarsity Press editors Jon Boyd and Rebecca Carhart. Jon's enduring support, enthusiasm, and editorial wisdom have been foundational for this project. Rebecca's inspiration and expertise have been especially instrumental in the final stages of the project. And a special thank you to the anonymous reviewers of the manuscript who provided insightful feedback and excellent suggestions for improvements.

I am grateful to Wheaton College for the sabbatical release time to conduct the research for this project. It is a privilege to serve under the gifted and empowering leadership of Provost Karen An-hwei Lee, Dean Sarah Hall, and Program Director Ki Chae. Heartfelt thanks to the Stacy and Timyan families, whose generous support provided the beautiful space for a writing retreat that was so timely and necessary to get this project off the ground.

Thank you to family, friends, and colleagues who expressed enthusiasm for this book and allowed me to quiz them about their own therapy experiences.

Our adult kids—Elise, Alec, and Allie—have especially inspired and challenged me to pursue justice, love, and mercy in all endeavors, including this one.

Finally, my deepest gratitude to my husband, Bob—life partner, cotherapist, and dive buddy—for his strong support of this project and his unwavering belief in the power of psychotherapy to bring about healing. It has been a joy to live out this calling together for the past forty years!

Getting Started

Welcome to the counseling journey! Whether you are new to the idea of therapy or a current counseling client looking to make the most of your experience, reading *The Client's Guide to Therapy* is a significant step in your personal growth journey. The following pages provide a modest and practical guide to the psychotherapy experience from start to finish. Integrating wisdom from scientific studies about effective counseling with real-life experiences from both counselors and counselees, this guide will address common questions and provide practical suggestions to guide you through each stage of therapy. My hope is that the information and examples in this book will demystify the process and break down any barriers that would keep those in need of counseling from seeking services.

For most new endeavors, whether for business or pleasure, we can find an abundance of guidebooks and resources to prepare us to make the most of the experience. One of my favorite parts of traveling is the process of trip planning. I greatly enjoy the hours spent poring over travel guides, examining online reviews, and collecting travel tips from knowledgeable guides. Accessing my inner travel nerd helps me to be well-informed about the opportunities and challenges that the destination brings and enables me to gain the most out of the traveling adventure.

As a psychologist in clinical practice for nearly forty years, I have been surprised by the scarcity of resources available to clients embarking on the counseling journey. The whole process of psychotherapy, from finding a therapist to knowing when you are finished, can be downright mystifying. Clients are often unsure about their role and how to partner with their therapist to cocreate a meaningful and effective therapy experience. An active and empowered client has the potential to gain the most from the counseling experience and ensure that psychotherapy is customized to address their real needs and concerns.

However, accurate information from a trustworthy guide can prove to be elusive, and it is easy to become overwhelmed by online searches as you try to determine what kind of therapy or therapist will address your needs. This task is incredibly daunting when you are in distress and need to find a therapist yesterday.

My favorite travel books include several features. Helpful guides provide great suggestions about not-to-miss sites and experiences, how to find a reputable guide, practical wisdom on navigating the basics (travel, food, money), and even what to do if things go wrong, for example, if you lose your passport (flee to the nearest embassy!). While this particular guidebook may not include inspiring travel photos, it will include snapshots of wisdom from insiders about how to gain the most from the counseling experience. It will also provide a map of sorts to help you know you are on the right track, make the most of challenging and illuminating detours, and determine when you have reached your destination.

Where Are We Headed?

Like any good travel guide, we will start with the highlights. Chapter one addresses the question, "Why should I consider therapy?" with an overview of the many reasons people seek counseling, the benefits that can be gained, and the common barriers that often keep people from much-needed treatment. Chapter two explores some practical questions about how to choose a therapist as a trustworthy guide for the counseling journey. Chapter three provides guidelines for beginning well and establishing a good working relationship with your therapist. Chapter four maps out the therapeutic process and describes how your personalized treatment plan is developed, while chapter five offers practical suggestions on how to gain the most from your counseling experience. In chapter six, we consider strategies for traversing the detours and impasses that inevitably occur during psychotherapy. The final chapter wraps up the stages of counseling with suggestions on how to know when you have reached the end of your therapy journey and how to end well.

If you are a prospective or current client with religious and spiritual commitments, this book aims to situate the process of psychological growth and transformation within God's overall plan for human flourishing and growth in spiritual maturity. Bringing our spiritual and religious values to the counseling and psychotherapy experience is of great importance and can imbue the process with deeper meaning and lasting impact. Each chapter includes a section on faith perspectives to encourage integrated psychological and spiritual growth throughout each stage of the counseling process.

In this book, I use the terms *counseling/counselor* and *psychotherapy/ therapist* interchangeably as I believe that the two approaches to mental health care are more alike than different in contemporary practice. Historically, distinctions have been made between the two, with *counseling* described as an approach that tends to be more wellness-focused by providing guidance and practical strategies that draw on client strengths, while *psychotherapy* has been described as a mental health treatment that helps clients identify the root causes of current symptoms and problems by providing an in-depth exploration of thoughts, feelings, and behaviors.[1] As I will discuss in chapter four, the primary difference between treatment approaches has more to do with the therapist's theoretical orientation than their professional identity. Thus, some counselors will be quite depth-oriented, while a psychotherapist or psychologist may also be strength-based and practically focused.

Throughout the book, I have attempted to balance valuable research findings with the very human and more subjective aspects of the therapeutic process. For example, we have learned quite a bit from research about the factors that lead to effective psychotherapy outcomes. This

---

[1]The American Counseling Association defines counseling as "a professional relationship that empowers diverse individuals, families and groups to accomplish mental health, wellness, education and career goals." "What Is Counseling?," American Counseling Association, www.counseling.org/mental-health-counseling/what-is-counseling#. The American Psychological Association defines psychotherapy as "any psychological service provided by a trained professional that primarily uses forms of communication and interaction to assess, diagnose, and treat dysfunctional emotional reactions, ways of thinking, and behavior patterns." "Psychotherapy," American Psychological Association, www .apa.org/topics/psychotherapy.

science of psychotherapy is invaluable for both clients and therapists as it highlights what aspects of the therapeutic process deserve particular emphasis. But it is equally valid that psychotherapy is a remarkably human encounter, fraught with all of the mystery and complexity of person-to-person interactions. I believe the relational dimensions of the therapy experience are among the most important, and I will seek to amplify both the client and therapist roles in fostering a solid therapy relationship of trust and collaboration as a necessary foundation for change and growth.

Why Read This Book?

In medicine, there is a practice called *role induction* that basically means educating patients about how they can play an active role in participating in a medical procedure to gain the maximum benefit. It makes good intuitive sense that people receiving health care services want to know what they are supposed to do to be a part of the healing process. For too long, patients in psychotherapy have been unnecessarily mystified by what they can do to gain the most from the counseling experience. I hope this book serves as a kind of role induction for anyone currently in or considering therapy. The fact that you have chosen to read this book shows that you are already the best kind of therapy client—motivated, curious, and proactive.

I also hope to let you in on the therapist's side of the experience to demystify the process further. I invite you to see us as fellow human beings and travelers who are also on our own mental health journey, indeed with our own set of issues and baggage. We have an ethical responsibility to manage our issues sufficiently so that the client's welfare will always precede. However, it is essential to the therapeutic process to bring our own authentic and flawed selves to the therapeutic encounter.

Ideally, my therapist colleagues will also find this guide to be a helpful and trustworthy resource for their clients, which will lead to stronger therapeutic collaboration and even better therapy outcomes. My aim is to pull back the curtain of the counseling process honestly and accurately as I try to put into words what we most want our clients to know. May this guide serve as an encouragement for you as you empower your clients to be trusted partners with you throughout their psychotherapy experience.

Throughout the book, you will find practical advice and helpful stories from my conversations with clients, colleagues, and friends and my own experiences as a therapy client. I have taken great care to change any identifying information to protect the anonymity of these persons and to seek permission when exact quotes are used.

Faith Perspectives: The Therapeutic Process as a Wilderness Journey

In this book I describe the counseling experience as a personal journey. But exactly what kind of travel adventure are we talking about? The rich symbolism of the wilderness journey provides a compelling vision for psychotherapy as an invitation to personal and spiritual transformation. Let's take a closer look at the wilderness journey and how this analogy offers a deeper understanding of what is possible through the counseling experience.

The wilderness experience as a metaphor for spiritual growth and personal transformation has inspired Jewish and Christian people throughout the centuries and provides us today with a meaningful way to understand the therapeutic endeavor. As recounted in Scripture, the wilderness as a place of transformation is a prominent theme in Judeo-Christian history. In the exodus narrative, the people of Israel escape captivity and are led by God to the Promised Land through a forty-year wilderness journey.[2] Leaving captivity as an enslaved community, the people of Israel follow their God-appointed leader, Moses, into the wilderness, where they learn through much trial and error to recognize their sins, forsake their idols, and depend on God's merciful provision of sustenance and law to guide their life together as a community. They also encounter miracles, failures, numerous setbacks, doubts, and infighting throughout their wanderings. In the wilderness, they learn

---

[2]The biblical narrative of the exodus journey can be found especially in the Old Testament books of Exodus, Numbers, and Deuteronomy.

individually and collectively to embrace their identity as the people of God. Sustained by hope in God's promised outcome, they persevere in the wilderness journey to find a new life in the Promised Land.

I invite you to consider that your counseling experience, too, can begin with a recognition of those places in your life where you are held captive, as familiar and sometimes comfortable as they might be. As you walk away from areas of personal imprisonment, you begin a journey into unknown territory, guided by your therapist but ultimately dependent on God's provision and protection. Through the process of therapy, you confront your idols, encounter setbacks, and face your doubts. Sometimes, you also question yourself (Do I want to go back to Egypt?), and you may wonder whether your therapist is a trustworthy guide. You also encounter some authentic "aha!" moments of insight or breakthrough where you glimpse the Promised Land. As you persevere, through God's grace, you arrive at a new destination as a psychologically healthier and spiritually more mature person than when you started.

The wilderness is the context where we can be transformed and our identity consolidated. A wise and experienced psychologist (who also happens to be my husband) describes the wilderness journey in this way: "The wilderness calls us out of the Egypt of our idolatrous attachments, supports us through the wilderness of shedding illusions, and stirs our longings for the promised land."[3]

The life of Jesus included a period at the beginning of his ministry where he was led by the Spirit into the wilderness and faced temptations by the devil (Matthew 4:1-11). Jesus' experience, as recounted in Scripture, sheds insight on the adversity that we as his followers will also confront in the wilderness. In his book *In the Name of Jesus*, Henri Nouwen examines the temptations Christians encounter today in light of Jesus' wilderness experience. As Nouwen points out, the temptations to be relevant, popular, and powerful can draw us away from the pursuit of God and the authentic Christian life. From a spiritual perspective, the

---

[3]Robert Watson and Michael Mangis, "Personhood, Spiritual Formation, and Intersubjectivity in the Tradition of the Desert Fathers and Mothers," in *On Being a Person: A Multidisciplinary Approach*, ed. Todd H. Speidell (Eugene, OR: Wipf & Stock, 2002), 54.

wilderness journey brings us face to face with our most hidden and sinful thoughts and desires as we are stripped of our standard methods of hiding and avoidance. We come to the end of our human abilities and recognize our complete dependence on the mercy and love of God for life and hope. Through trials and tribulations, we confront the stark realization that we have nothing to offer others except our own vulnerable and broken selves.[4]

Recently, my husband and I took a pilgrimage journey in Scotland, following St. Conan's Way through the Highlands and the Isle of Mull to the holy island of Iona. We did our best to prepare for the journey by getting in shape, packing our backpacks with supplies, and studying ordnance maps of the Scottish Highlands. Inevitably, we encountered challenges and detours along the way that were painfully humbling and difficult yet offered holy moments of grace and revelation. As we faced our limitations, human frailties, and shortcomings, we grew in our dependence on God's protection and provision through the kindness of strangers. For example, a sympathetic couple from Glasgow took pity on us as we struggled up an especially grueling hill and loaded us into their car with our backpacks and muddy boots for a ride to the top. And we will never forget the woman who pulled over to us in her car during a spirit-dampening Scottish downpour and assured us there was a warm and dry community center with tea and cake just ahead that would welcome us. Looking back, these moments of vulnerable dependence on God's care through others were as deeply meaningful as reaching our destination. Wilderness experiences can be transformative as we step out of our comfort zone to rely on the love of God and the mercy of others.

In many ways, the counseling journey can be considered your own mental health pilgrimage as you travel the length and breadth of your soul to discover more of God and yourself. Psalm 84:5-7 says it best, expressing my hope and prayer for you as you begin this book:

---

[4]Henri Nouwen, *In the Name of Jesus: Reflections on Christian Leadership* (New York: Crossroad, 1989).

Blessed are those whose strength is in you,
  whose hearts are set on pilgrimage.
As they pass through the Valley of Baka,[5]
  they make it a place of springs;
  the autumn rains also cover it with pools.
They go from strength to strength,
  till each appears before God in Zion.

---

[5]"Valley of weeping" in some Bible translations.

1

How Can Psychotherapy Help?

Contemplating the Counseling Journey

*I've had your name for a couple of years, but
recently, my depression has gotten worse.*

*I feel I can't go on like this in my work. A colleague
told me I have all the signs of burnout, and I need to
figure out how I got here and how I can recover.*

*There are some issues from my growing-up years that I know I need
to work on before getting married and starting my own family.*

*I'm struggling to understand where God is
in the midst of all of this anxiety.*

<small>EXAMPLES OF CLIENT STATEMENTS FROM
INITIAL PHONE INQUIRIES ABOUT PSYCHOTHERAPY</small>

Every counseling journey begins with hope. Something in your life
is not how it should be, and you long for change. You may hope for
relief from the nagging distress of painful thoughts and feelings. Or
you are reeling in the aftermath of a traumatic experience or loss and
hoping for someone to help you find your footing again. Maybe you
know something is out of alignment in your life, relationships, or career
and wish for the time and space to figure things out. Perhaps you long
for a life free from destructive habits or addictive behaviors and need
a trusted ally to help set you on the path to recovery. The many challenges encountered during a lifetime bring each one of us to that
moment where we recognize that we need help. Seeking help from

others is an act of *hope* that we do not have to struggle alone in our present suffering.

When the inevitable difficulties in life occur, a psychotherapist can be an invaluable companion and guide for the journey toward health and wholeness. As you bring your problems to a mental health professional, you develop a new and different perspective on your issues that removes obstacles and creates a pathway forward for both acceptance and change. In the context of a confidential and trusting counseling relationship, you make connections, gain insights, and slowly but surely begin to move steadily along the pathway to restoration and transformation. Psychotherapy can be quite an illuminating journey where, in addition to dealing with pain and suffering, you deeply explore life questions about who you are and where you are going. These essential questions often get pushed aside in the busyness of everyday living.

People seek counseling and psychotherapy for many different reasons and with a variety of goals in mind. Some examples include:

- for help with emotional difficulties stemming from a loss, transition, or crisis
- to improve relationships with family, friends, or colleagues
- to address professional burnout and career concerns
- for parenting support and help related to concerns for a child or adolescent
- to cope with intrusive or distressing thoughts
- to break free of addictive or compulsive behaviors
- to deal with problems in self-esteem and identity
- to address spiritual or existential struggles and make meaning of suffering
- for growth in self-awareness and understanding
- to address long-standing challenges and unresolved issues from the past
- to accept those aspects of ourselves and our circumstances that may not be changeable
- at the request of a friend, family member, or employer

When a client comes to me for psychotherapy, I often find that their most urgent question is this: "If I invest my hope in the counseling process and in you as my therapist, can you help me? When I begin to lose hope, can I borrow your hope that things can truly get better?" The answer to this essential question is an unequivocal yes. As therapists, we honor this investment of hope from our clients as a sacred trust. We recognize just how hard our clients have worked to solve problems on their own and know how difficult it is to hold on to hope for the possibility of change when so many attempts have been unsuccessful. Our commitment to you is to be a trustworthy companion on your journey toward wholeness and healing as we draw from our professional training and personal experiences to provide informed guidance.

Ultimately, the journey toward health begins with the recognition that we do not have to travel alone in our quest to address the problems in our lives. Psychotherapy brings the hope of change and the promise of a trusted companion and guide on the pathway to emotional, relational, and spiritual health. The question, "Why should I consider psychotherapy?" comes down to this: *Where do I hope for change in my life?*

What Is Psychotherapy, and Why Should You Consider It?

Counseling and psychotherapy are professional services that provide effective treatment of emotional, relational, and psychological distress to improve mental health and enhance overall well-being. Provided by a licensed professional who meets the educational and experience requirements of their state and national accrediting body, psychotherapy applies scientifically based principles to relieve psychological symptoms in the context of a confidential, supportive relationship. Counseling can include individual, group, couple, and family treatment. While there are many distinctive mental health disciplines, all counselors are committed to ethical principles and standards of practice that regulate the profession and ensure the client receives effective treatment from a qualified professional. Psychotherapy is considered a medical intervention and is covered by most health insurance plans when there is a reimbursable mental health diagnosis.

What exactly do therapists do to help? Generally, we work collaboratively with clients to remove obstacles to growth and change through active listening, offering support, promoting insight, providing objective observations, offering psychoeducation, and teaching coping skills. In addition, we will help clients change their thought patterns, provide strategies for behavior change, and deepen their understanding of their emotions. Counselors are equipped to help clients realize problematic relational patterns, deal with traumatic experiences, work through grief reactions, and find meaning in times of suffering. Clients' gains in counseling will generalize to other areas of their lives and prepare them to cope effectively with future difficulties.

As a psychologist, I believe there are many compelling reasons to embark on the counseling journey, and I highlight the top five benefits of psychotherapy in this next section. In brief, psychotherapy can lead to significant improvements in health, quality of life, spiritual vitality, and the ability to deal with life's challenges. Its positive effects are strongly supported by scientific studies. Let's look more closely at each of these benefits.

Reason 1: Psychotherapy improves mental health. In any journey, we begin by contemplating the destination. I have described why people pursue counseling, but to what end? What *is* mental health, and why is it essential for our lives? Simply put, mental health involves our emotional, intellectual, behavioral, and social functioning and well-being. When we are mentally healthy, we can generally manage the day-to-day activities involved in making decisions, using our abilities to engage in meaningful tasks, pursue our goals, and connect with others in mutually supportive relationships. We can cope adequately with day-to-day stressors and roll with life's changes when inevitable difficulties arise. The World Health Organization offers this succinct definition of mental health: "A state of mental well-being that enables people to cope with the stresses of life, to realize their abilities, to learn well and work well, and to contribute to their communities."[1]

Maintaining mental health throughout our lives is an elusive task, however. Estimates are that over half of all adults will experience psychological symptoms consistent with a mental illness at some point during their lifetime.[2] Thus, for most of us, the question is not *whether* but *when* we find ourselves in need of psychotherapy.

Mental health problems and symptoms are common to the human experience and exist on a continuum from expected emotional distress in response to stressful situations and losses (grief, for example) to severe mental illnesses such as chronic mood disorders or psychotic disorders. The Covid-19 pandemic has raised awareness of the debilitating effects of mental illness on overall health and human functioning. Recent surveys have identified a significant increase in reported mental health concerns in the wake of the pandemic, with over 40 percent of adults in the United States reporting that they are struggling with anxiety, depression, trauma symptoms, suicidal thoughts, or substance abuse, compared to the 11 percent of adults reporting symptoms in 2019.[3] The increasing need for postpandemic services combined with diminishing access to mental health care takes a significant emotional and financial toll on individuals, families, and communities, contributing to the emerging mental health crisis.[4] We owe it to ourselves and those we

---

[1] World Health Organization, "World Mental Health Report: Transforming Mental Health for All," World Health Organization, June 16, 2022, 8, www.who.int/publications/i/item/9789240049338.

[2] Ronald C. Kessler et al., "Lifetime Prevalence and Age-of-Onset Distributions of Mental Disorders in the World Health Organization's World Mental Health Survey Initiative," *World Psychiatry: Official Journal of the World Psychiatric Association* 6, no. 3 (October 2007): 168-76, https://pubmed.ncbi.nlm.nih.gov/18188442/.

[3] Mark E. Czeisler, Rashon I. Lane, and Emiko Petrosky, "Mental Health, Substance Use, and Suicidal Ideation During the COVID-19 Pandemic—United States," *Morbidity and Mortality Weekly Report* 69, no. 32 (2020): 1049-57, https://doi.org/10.15585/mmwr.mm6932a1; National Center for Health Statistics, "Early Release of Selected Mental Health Estimates Based on Data from the January–June 2019 National Health Interview Survey," Center for Disease Control and Prevention, 2020, www.cdc.gov/nchs/data/nhis/earlyrelease/ERmentalhealth-508.pdf.

[4] "Reducing the Economic Burden of Unmet Mental Health Needs," The White House, 2022, www.whitehouse.gov/cea/written-materials/2022/05/31/reducing-the-economic-burden-of-unmet-mental-health-needs/.

love to stay informed about the signs, symptoms, and causes of mental illness and to know how and when to seek treatment.

What causes mental illness? Scientific research has closely examined the risk factors that contribute to the development of mental health symptoms. Most often, there is no single or straightforward cause for mental health problems. Instead, our mental health is influenced by several interacting factors:[5]

- our biology, which includes genetics and family history, chronic medical conditions, substance abuse, sleep difficulties, and nutrition
- our psychology, including any childhood traumas, adverse life experiences, or chronic stress
- social and economic stressors, including social isolation, poverty, experiences of marginalization or racism, and lack of access to resources
- spiritual factors, including existential isolation, meaninglessness, feeling inherently flawed or punished by God

I have found that many clients enter therapy with the expectation that they can pinpoint the exact cause of their current problems and symptoms. The challenge is that many psychological issues are multi-determined and multifaceted. Therefore, it can be difficult to identify one specific trigger or cause. The question, "Why are these symptoms developing now?" can be a fruitful area for exploration and lead to the identification of environmental triggers and risk factors that contribute to current psychological struggles. For clients, understanding "How did I get here?" can bring relief and help us anticipate future risk factors to pay attention to.

The flip side of *risk* factors is that we also possess biopsychosocial and spiritual *protective* factors that can mitigate the development of mental illness. Protective factors include good overall physical health, social support, positive environmental resources, and healthy religious and moral

---

[5]Marcelo Saad, Roberta de Medeiros, and Amanda Cristina Mosini, "Are We Ready for a True Biopsychosocial-Spiritual Model? The Many Meanings of 'Spiritual,'" *Medicines (Basel)* 4, no. 79 (October 2017): 1-2, doi:10.3390/medicines4040079.

belief systems.[6] As therapists, we are very interested in not only assessing what is wrong but also identifying client strengths and protective factors, as they become essential resources for clients to continue to draw on throughout the journey toward improved mental health. I recall one family I worked with who checked about every box for risk factors and environmental stressors. However, their open and supportive communication with one another, combined with an astounding sense of humor, made it possible for them to endure substantive hardship with minimal lasting mental health effects. Clients will often express surprise and relief as we spend time in therapy identifying their protective factors and the sources of their resilience. Psychotherapy does not just focus on problems but also seeks to understand how people can survive and thrive amid adverse experiences.

A client once described the benefits of understanding their risk and protective factors in this way:

> It was important to me to figure out the causes of my panic attacks and why they started when they did. As we put my history together, my attitude shifted from shame and self-condemnation to the realization that anyone in my shoes would have been overwhelmed given the circumstances. I am relieved to have a toolbox of coping skills I've learned through therapy to help me in the future.

The counseling journey affirms the essential importance of good mental health as therapists and clients work together to alleviate distressing symptoms, identify risk factors, and highlight protective factors that can strengthen resilience for the future. The destination of the counseling journey is improved mental health, which is essential to every other aspect of our lives.

Reason 2: Counseling enhances quality of life and sense of purpose. "What is the good life?" is a question at the heart of what it means to be human. This topic transcends the discipline of psychology and has engaged philosophers, theologians, and leading thinkers throughout history. It is also a highly personal question that each of us must grapple

---

[6]Saad, de Medeiros, and Mosini, "Are We Ready?"

with as our response may determine our sense of well-being, life meaning, and happiness. A desire to minimize pain and maximize pleasure is part of the human condition. But questions about the good life take us beyond simple hedonism to something more profound: Who am I, and what is my purpose? What gifts or character strengths am I endowed with that can be developed and used for the greater good? What can I give to the world that will provide my life with meaning and purpose? Psychotherapy offers an ideal context to step away from our everyday routines and delve deeper into these fundamentally human questions that are essential for our quality of life and sense of purpose.

Our sense of well-being is closely connected to our personal take on the good life and how we assess our progress toward obtaining this elusive goal. The Berkeley Well-Being Institute offers this definition: "Well-being is defined as a sense of health and vitality that arises from your thoughts, emotions, actions, and experiences. When we have well-being, we feel happy, healthy, socially connected, and purposeful most of the time."[7] Our subjective feelings of well-being are one aspect of our overall mental health, and improving well-being is a primary goal of psychotherapy. As one of my clients exclaimed, "I feel like I am going through the motions of my life but not really living. There *must* be more than this. I just want to feel like myself again!"

For over 150 years, the discipline of psychology has sought answers to essential human questions through academic study, rigorous research, and clinical practice. While the primary focus of much of psychology's history has been the study of mental illness, a more recent emphasis in the past twenty years has been on the science of human flourishing, aptly named *positive psychology*. The rich theories, research, and practices that positive psychologists have generated have greatly informed our scientific understanding of essential topics such as happiness, resilience, character strengths, relationship health, and well-being. Leading positive psychologist Martin Seligman uses the acronym PERMA to describe the

---

[7]Tchiki Davis, "Well-Being: Definition, Types, and Psychology," Berkely Well-Being Institute, accessed September 23, 2022, www.berkeleywellbeing.com/what-is-well-being.html.

components of well-being: positive emotions, engagement, relationships, meaning, and achievement.[8] Positive psychologists conduct research and develop specific interventions and practices to help people develop daily habits leading to greater flourishing. I find these flourishing practices to be quite helpful when working with clients who are experiencing exhaustion and burnout and are ready to recalibrate their lives.

Many psychological theories, including positive psychology, assume that humans possess an innate motivation for psychological growth, health, and secure relational attachment to others. Just like our physical bodies are oriented toward health and attempt to heal by producing symptoms (i.e., fever, pain) to rid the body of illness, psychological symptoms may also indicate that something is wrong that our body and brain are attempting to heal. A major benefit of psychotherapy is the alleviation of psychological symptoms so that our natural inclination toward growth and health can develop. Psychotherapy, then, is not just about addressing problems. It also helps us improve our well-being and quality of life so that we can live, love, learn, and contribute meaningfully to society.

Reason 3: Psychological growth contributes to spiritual vitality. Our individual worldview and personal values greatly affect our vision of the good life and how it can be achieved. A theological and biblical framework views human beings as created in God's image and for a relationship with God, who has "set eternity in the human heart" (Ecclesiastes 3:11). Existential and spiritual struggles can contribute to the development of psychological symptoms. Psychotherapist and spiritual writer Thomas Moore writes that we must honor these symptoms as the "voice of the soul."[9] One client described their experience this way: "A turning point in my therapy was when we figured out that my tension and irritability at work stemmed from losing my vocational dreams when I missed out on my desired promotion. Why would God let that happen? I think my unresolved anger and loss were literally making me sick!"

---

[8]Martin Seligman, *Flourish* (New York: Simon & Schuster, 2013).
[9]Thomas Moore, *Care of the Soul* (New York: Harper Perennial, 1992), 3.

For many Christian clients, one of the important benefits of counseling is the opportunity to make sense of our difficulties in the context of our faith commitments. Suffering affects our relationship with God and often triggers spiritual and theological questions. Counselors help clients wrestle faithfully with these questions in a manner consistent with their value commitments. Therapists support clients' exploration of questions and doubts while encouraging them to stay connected with their faith communities for guidance and spiritual resources.

From a faith perspective, I believe that God desires our spiritual vitality and can use the process of counseling and psychotherapy to eliminate obstacles to growth, health, and relational connection. Ultimately, we glorify God when we can bring our healthiest selves, that is, who he created us to be, to living and loving. We can see God at work through the process of counseling and psychotherapy as he helps us discern the barriers that exist to a fuller and more God-honoring life. An honest and courageous examination of our thoughts, feelings, and behaviors, while sometimes daunting, also leads us further along in our spiritual journey and ultimately helps us, by the grace of God, to remove the barriers to loving God and our neighbor. We can bring our faith commitments and spiritual practices into each phase of the counseling process, as I will invite you to do in the following chapters. I am a firm believer that counseling is good for the soul.

Reason 4: Psychotherapy strengthens our ability to deal with inevitable life challenges and find meaning and purpose in times of suffering. It is often a difficult realization that even the good life involves periods of loss, suffering, and hardship. "Where is God in my suffering and pain?" is a constant question that people of faith must wrestle with throughout our lives. When the inevitable times of suffering occur, our view of ourselves, others, and the world is often called into question. Times of transition, loss, and trauma can challenge our most cherished beliefs and values.

The human impulse to avoid suffering can create more significant problems and symptoms. Over time, these coping strategies can develop into problematic ways of thinking, feeling, and behaving that detract from our overall mental health and well-being. For example, a typical response following a traumatic event is to adopt strategies to avoid any situation that elicits memories or reminders of the event. These avoidance strategies, however, often create problems as more situations are avoided in self-protection, and our world can begin to constrict. I remember how, following a car accident, I began to avoid driving altogether as getting behind the wheel brought feelings of anxiety and memories of the accident. It was only through sitting with the very uncomfortable feelings of fear and anxiety behind the wheel that I was able to begin driving again and resume my everyday life. Psychotherapy provides a supportive context for clients to do the necessary work of tolerating distress and suffering so that healing can occur.

I worked with a client who requested help in dealing with a sudden onset of feelings of hopelessness and despair about her life that were affecting her ability to work at her job. In her mid-fifties, she described herself as a naturally optimistic person, and she was mystified about why she was experiencing such pessimistic thoughts, anger at God, and debilitating feelings of dysphoria. As we explored these symptoms, we discovered that the onset of symptoms occurred shortly after the sudden death of a dear friend, a significant loss that she had not yet processed. As she engaged in the difficult work of mourning the loss of her friend and giving voice to the spiritual questions and struggles that had emerged, the client's symptoms began to abate, and her characteristic optimism started to reemerge.

Often, experiences of suffering lay bare our spiritual questions and struggles that have no easy answers. Voicing these deeply felt spiritual and existential concerns with a trusted therapist as a faithful companion can move us further along the pathway to finding meaning in our suffering. The concept of posttraumatic growth is used to describe the process of positive change and transformation that can occur following a significant stressor or challenge.[10] As Romans 5:3-4 reminds us, "We know that suffering produces perseverance; perseverance, character;

---

[10]Richard Tedeshi and Lawrence G. Calhoun, *Posttraumatic Growth: Conceptual Foundation and Empirical Evidence* (Philadelphia: Lawrence Erlbaum Associates, 2004).

and character, hope." Finding meaning, purpose, or opportunity for growth in our suffering can boost coping and resilience for present and future struggles. One of my clients described her desire for posttraumatic growth in this compelling way: "I want to be changed by these present difficulties—I don't want to waste this suffering!"

Reason 5: It works! If the reasons above have not yet convinced you that psychotherapy is a valuable and worthwhile endeavor, consider the simple fact that psychotherapy works as a reason to give it a try. Researchers have amassed a significant amount of scientific evidence over the years that demonstrates the benefits of psychotherapy.[11] We will discuss the findings in greater detail in future chapters, but here are some of the highlights:

- Half of all clients report a significant decrease in their mental health symptoms by session eight of psychotherapy.

- This percentage increases to 75 percent of clients reporting significant improvements at the twenty-six-session mark.[12]

- Positive changes made through psychotherapy are maintained, and improvements continue even after therapy is concluded.

- Psychotherapy improves overall physical health, including decreases in illness and disability.

- Improvements in functioning in the workplace are an outcome of psychotherapy for many people.

- Psychotherapy leads to improvements in relationships for individuals, couples, and families.[13]

In 2013, the American Psychological Association passed this milestone resolution affirming the effectiveness of psychotherapy based on decades of research:

---

[11] American Psychological Association, "Recognition of Psychotherapy Effectiveness," *Psychotherapy* 50, no. 1 (2013): 102-9, doi:10.1037/a0030276.

[12] Kenneth I. Howard, S. Mark Kopta, Merton S. Krause, and David E. Orlinsky, "The Dose-Effect Relationship in Psychotherapy," *American Psychologist* 41, no. 2 (1986): 159-64, https://psycnet.apa.org/record/1986-17818-001?doi=1.

[13] American Psychological Association, "Recognition of Psychotherapy Effectiveness."

Be It Resolved that, as a healing practice and professional service, psychotherapy is effective and highly cost-effective. In controlled trials and in clinical practice, psychotherapy results in benefits that markedly exceed those experienced by individuals who need mental health services but do not receive psychotherapy. Consequently, psychotherapy should be included in the health care system as an established evidence-based practice.[14]

For clients, keeping these proven benefits in mind can provide hope and confidence throughout the counseling journey.

DOES EVERYONE NEED THERAPY?

As the benefits of psychotherapy have become widely known, it has become more acceptable and perhaps even the norm to see a counselor for help with personal growth goals in addition to dealing with life difficulties. While this decrease in stigma is an improvement, it raises the question: Does everyone need therapy?

In response, I defer to the National Institute for Mental Health guidelines for determining whether you need professional help for mental health symptoms.[a] The first step is to assess how your symptoms interfere with day-to-day functioning. For mild mental health symptoms that have been present for less than two weeks, the National Institute for Mental Health recommends that the first plan of action is to make use of self-care approaches to help with symptoms. These strategies include talking to a friend, pursuing social interactions, exercising, improving sleep, and practicing meditation and mindfulness. An example of mild symptoms would be if you are feeling a little anxious or down but can still function in your daily life (i.e., work, study, or care for others).

If the symptoms persist beyond two weeks, worsen, or interfere with your daily functioning, you are encouraged to seek out professional help by contacting a mental health or medical provider. Examples of more severe symptoms include but are not limited to thoughts of self-harm or death, difficulty getting out of bed, inability to work or go to school, loss of concentration, significant weight loss or gain, inability to sleep, or loss of interest or pleasure in daily activities. When in doubt, consult your health care provider to determine the best course of action.

---

[14]American Psychological Association, "Recognition of Psychotherapy Effectiveness."

It is vital that you seek immediate help if you are having current thoughts of hurting yourself or someone else by going to your local emergency room, calling 911, or calling or texting the Suicide and Crisis Line at 988. Outside the United States, you can find listings of crisis hotlines by country through the International Association of Suicide Prevention at www.iasp.info/suicidalthoughts/.

[a]U.S. Department of Health and Human Services, "My Mental Health: Do I Need Help?," National Institutes of Health NIH publication no. 22-MH-8134, accessed September 1, 2023, www.nimh.nih.gov/health/publications/my-mental-health-do-i-need-help.

Common Barriers to Accessing Mental Health Care

Despite the proven benefits of psychotherapy, many people who experience significant psychological symptoms find it difficult to access the very help that could alleviate their distress. One extensive study found delays on average of eleven years after symptoms occurred before clients sought treatment from a mental health professional.[15] What are the barriers to mental health care, and how can we address them?

Affordability. The cost of psychological services remains a significant barrier for many, particularly uninsured or underinsured individuals and families. Figuring out how to use health insurance benefits to pay for mental health treatment can be daunting, but it has the potential to increase the affordability of services significantly. Insurers have been slow to reimburse treatment of behavioral health and addictions at the same level as other medical care despite the evidence that improved mental health positively affects overall health. Fortunately, important legislation has provided support for consumer rights. The Mental Health Parity Law established in 2008 requires insurance companies to reimburse mental health care at the same rate as other medical treatments and applies to many health plans.[16] However, high deductibles for health care or reduced coverage for out-of-network providers can pose a significant financial burden to accessing mental health care.

[15]Philip S. Wang, Patricia A. Berglund, Mark Olfson, and Ronald C. Kessler, "Delays in Initial Treatment Contact After First Onset of a Mental Disorder," *Health Service Research* 39, no. 2 (2004): 393-415, doi:10.1111/j.1475-6773.2004.00234.x.
[16]"Does Your Insurance Cover Mental Health Services?," American Psychological Association, May 14, 2014, www.apa.org/topics/managed-care-insurance/parity-guide.

For the uninsured or underinsured, community mental health services are available in most geographic areas, where clients are offered services on a sliding scale based on income. Some community counseling centers will have a waiting list, and it is advisable to call to get yourself on the list as soon as you begin to consider mental health services, even if you continue to pursue other treatment options. Another good choice for affordable services is to access counseling through a university-affiliated training clinic, where counselors-in-training provide psychotherapy under the supervision of licensed professionals.

Mental health professionals can often work with clients to make their services affordable and accessible. Agreeing on a sustainable financial arrangement is an important first step in finding a therapist. Some therapists are able to bill insurance on the client's behalf, and clients will then pay their deductible and copayment at the time of service. Other counselors use a fee-for-service model and request that their clients pay at the time of services, then provide the documentation for clients to submit claims to their insurance company or employer health spending account. Many providers offer limited sliding-scale services based on client income and financial need. If affordability is a barrier to receiving needed mental health care, I encourage you to ask prospective therapists about the availability of reduced fees and payment plans.

TIPS FOR ACCESSING HEALTH INSURANCE COVERAGE FOR PSYCHOTHERAPY

Many insurance plans include some coverage for medically necessary treatment of mental and behavioral health issues. Researching your coverage before making that first call to a therapist can result in significant cost savings and help you narrow down available options and choices. Contact your insurance company using the phone number on your insurance card, and be sure to check to see if there is a different number for behavioral health or mental health services. You can also access information about your health coverage online or through your employer's human resources department. While every insurance plan is different, there are some general questions to remember as you explore your policy's coverage of mental health treatment.

Do I need a referral for behavioral or mental health services? Some policies require you to obtain a referral from your primary care provider for treatment by a mental health professional, similar to other kinds of specialist care. Your provider or insurer may ask you some questions about your symptoms and day-to-day functioning to determine whether a referral is medically necessary.

Is there a difference between in-network versus out-of-network coverage? Your plan may offer different reimbursement rates if you see a provider in their network, but it may also cover some out-of-network services. Inquire about any differences in coverage. Request access to the list of in-network providers in your area. Some clients may prefer to have greater flexibility in choosing their preferred therapist and opt out of the network, while others will value the cost savings from seeing an in-network provider.

What are my out-of-pocket costs? It is important to inquire about anticipated out-of-pocket costs for services. Many plans require participants to meet an out-of-pocket deductible for medical care before their reimbursement kicks in. Once the deductible is met, there may be a copayment for services. Your insurance company can verify your benefits and provide information on these costs. Many employers have benefits such as flexible spending accounts or health savings accounts that allow employees to make pretax paycheck contributions that can then be used to pay for deductible and copay healthcare costs.

Will my counselor bill my insurance company directly for services? Your mental health provider may be able to assist you with the insurance billing process, and you can certainly inquire. Some therapy offices are set up to verify client insurance, provide an estimate of costs, and bill the insurance company, which will reimburse the provider directly. Other therapy offices are fee-for-service only, where the client is responsible for payment for services and then submitting an invoice for reimbursement to their insurance company.

Are there any drawbacks to using health insurance to pay for psychotherapy? The pros and cons of using health insurance to pay for counseling are worth considering. For many clients, insurance increases the affordability of psychotherapy, offers a streamlined process for billing and reimbursement, and ensures that providers are appropriately credentialed and meet the insurer's requirements. However, other clients may forgo the use of health insurance and prefer a fee-for-service arrangement that can provide greater privacy, flexibility, and the freedom to choose a provider that best meets their needs and preferences.

You are not alone if you need help navigating your insurance coverage for psychotherapy. However, my word of advice is to be persistent in getting your questions answered so you can make an informed decision.

Access. It is sometimes difficult to know where to begin to find good mental health care. Physicians, employers, educators, and community or religious leaders are often the first resources whom individuals turn to in times of emotional distress, and these professionals can provide referrals to a qualified mental health professional or treatment center. People who live outside major metropolitan areas, especially in rural areas, may encounter a greater scarcity of resources for mental health treatment. The availability of telehealth options has increased accessibility for many clients, and the client and therapist can assess together whether this modality is appropriate and effective for the client's presenting concerns.

Another challenge related to access is the lack of representation among mental health providers for clients from diverse and marginalized groups. Many clients want a therapist who understands and respects their cultural and community context. Finding a therapist who shares essential components of the client's experience adds a layer of complexity to finding and accessing the right therapist. Asking trusted friends, professionals, and colleagues for names of therapists who would be a good fit is often the most effective strategy. Prospective clients can also use online therapist directories that enable therapist searches by geographic location, therapist characteristics, and areas of specialization. Stay tuned for chapter two, where we will explore in greater detail how to access mental health treatment and where to find a therapist.

Since the pandemic, the demand for counseling services has grown considerably. You may find the right therapist and treatment option, only to learn that the therapist or treatment center has a waiting list. Do not give up! Practice good self-care strategies and seek out the support of friends, family, community leaders, and self-help resources while waiting for a therapist's opening. Be sure not to delay in contacting your medical provider if your symptoms worsen, or seek out immediate help (call 911, the 988 trauma line, or go to the emergency room) if you have thoughts of suicide or self-harm.

Social stigma and myths about psychotherapy. Despite the increased acceptance of counseling and psychotherapy as a normative life experience, many adults continue to refrain from seeking services due to stigma. Stigma is "a set of negative and often unfair beliefs that a society or group of people have about something."[17] Negative beliefs about those who experience psychological symptoms or receive mental health care can act as a deterrent to seeking needed services. Often, these negative beliefs are shared by others in our cultural group or community and can persist despite education to the contrary.

The media has shaped how we envision the therapy experience, providing depictions of those seeking therapy and the therapists who help them. While psychotherapy in the media can help normalize the act of seeking help for psychological problems, the media can also perpetuate myths and misconceptions. Negative (and untrue) beliefs that contribute to social stigma toward psychotherapy can include false beliefs that people who seek counseling are crazy or weak, for example. Some cultural norms may include the belief that sharing our problems with anyone outside the family or community is shameful or wrong. Religious communities can convey the message that the need for counseling is an indication of spiritual immaturity or insufficient trust in God. These messages could not be further from the truth, as it requires faith, hope, and courage to recognize and act on the need for help.

I am deeply grieved by the social stigma around mental health issues that continues to persist in many communities and poses a barrier for some clients to seek out the counseling they desperately need. However, I believe we have come a long way toward correcting these misperceptions about mental health issues in the church and society. It is encouraging to see community and religious leaders proactively reducing stigma by openly sharing about their own mental health journey and advocating for the benefits of effective treatment.

Stoic endurance and invulnerability. A common barrier to recognizing the need for help is the belief that we can (and should) deal with problems independently and without complaint. The notion of disclosing our feelings and concerns to another, specifically someone

---

[17]"Stigma," The Britannica Dictionary, accessed September 23, 2022, www.britannica.com /dictionary/stigma.

outside our community, is antithetical to many cultural norms, including those in my rural Midwestern background. When difficulties arise, we are taught to pull ourselves up by our bootstraps and soldier on alone or turn to helpers in our own community. I remember as a college student telling my parents about my professional aspiration to become a psychologist, only to have them exclaim with horror, "But we don't even believe in psychology!" Fortunately, the discipline of psychology exists, whether we believe in it or not, with growing acceptance in most communities of the value of counseling and psychotherapy services.

For those who value stoic endurance and invulnerability, admitting problems and asking for help may evoke a sense of embarrassment and shame. Shame is an internalized stigma that can hinder seeking counseling services. We may believe our problems indicate that we are defective at our core and beyond help or redemption. Valuing invulnerability, we may fear it will be too humiliating and painful to reveal our private sufferings to another human being and ask for help. The truth, however, is that seeking help through counseling indicates maturity and hope as we begin to see our suffering in a more truthful and realistic light as evidence of our common humanity rather than a personal failure.

Additional barriers for marginalized groups. Issues of affordability, access, and social stigma are magnified for clients from groups historically underserved by mental health care. According to the Centers for Disease Control, people from racial and ethnic minority groups have experienced more severe mental health impacts from the Covid-19 pandemic compared to the non-Hispanic white population yet face significant barriers in accessing professional services for treatable and preventable mental health issues. These barriers include financial challenges (including lack of insurance or insufficient insurance), difficulty finding diverse providers, inadequate cultural competence among mental health professionals, and social stigma related to mental illness.[18] Marginalized groups face the additional obstacle of mistrust in the mental health

---

[18]"Prioritizing Minority Mental Health," Centers for Disease Control and Prevention, June 27, 2023, www.cdc.gov/minority-health/features/minority-mental-health.html.

system associated with the risk of discrimination, bias, and stigmatization in diagnosis and treatment.[19] A conversation I had with a client illustrates this tension, as they shared with me, "Don't take this personally; it is just harder to open up to a therapist from the same culture and religion that has been oppressive to me all my life."

Health equity, according to the World Health Organization, is a fundamental human right and starts with acknowledging and addressing the obstacles to healthcare access for many groups.[20] It is imperative that all clients, particularly those from historically marginalized groups, have access to mental health care that is culturally competent, non-discriminatory, and respectful of diverse client experiences and perspectives. However, it can be challenging for many clients to find a therapist who understands their experience. Historically marginalized groups that may find difficulties accessing mental health care include but are not limited to racial and ethnic minority groups, low-income families, sexual and gender minority groups, and clients with differential abilities (including neurodiverse individuals).[21]

Just, fair, and equal access to quality mental health care are ethical imperatives for the mental health professions. For example, the American Psychological Association's "Ethical Principles of Psychologists" articulates a primary commitment to justice in the provision of research, education, assessment, and treatment, stating, "Psychologists recognize that fairness and justice entitle all persons to access to and benefit from the contributions of psychology and to equal quality in the processes, procedures, and services being conducted by psychologists."[22] Accredited graduate training programs for mental health professionals require students to learn best practices for

---

[19]Francesca Mongelli, Penelope Georgakopoulos, and Michele T. Pato, "Challenges and Opportunities to Meet the Mental Health Needs of Underserved and Disenfranchised Populations in the United States," *Focus* 18, no. 1 (January 2020): 16-24, doi:10.1176/appi.focus.20190028.

[20]"Health Equity," World Health Organization, accessed September 20, 2022, www.who.int/health-topics/health-equity#tab=tab_1.

[21]Mongelli, Georgakopoulos, and Pato, "Challenges and Opportunities."

[22]"Ethical Principles of Psychologists and Code of Conduct," American Psychological Association, 2017, www.apa.org/ethics/code.

diversity competence and how to provide culturally competent mental health care. A skilled therapist will seek to understand and address the demographic differences between themselves and their clients toward establishing strong therapy relationships.

However, as therapists, we also have our weak points and unconscious biases, which require us to embrace cultural humility, self-awareness, and openness to feedback from our clients about the aspects of their lives and culture we are missing. In many ways, all therapy relationships are crosscultural encounters, and it is a mistake for therapists to assume we know our clients based on demographic similarities or differences. I am constantly grateful for the patience and forbearance of my clients as we figure out together how to deepen awareness of our differences to form a therapy relationship of trust and mutual understanding of all our unique dimensions of diversity.

What if I've Tried Therapy Before?

If you have tried counseling before and it didn't seem to help, do not lose hope. There are many therapists and types of therapies, and sometimes it takes a few tries to find the right fit. Occasionally, I work with clients who were disappointed by their past experiences in therapy. Identifying what did not go well in their previous therapy helped us make the necessary adjustments to our own work together so that a more successful counseling experience could occur.

Sometimes, the lack of a good fit between the client and therapist interferes with the development of trust. As we have discussed previously, the client and therapist do not have to share the same diversity characteristics to work well together, but there does have to be curiosity and willingness to explore differences so the client can feel seen, understood, and safe in the context of the relationship.

As you think about another course of counseling, it may be advantageous to consider a different approach to therapy than you experienced previously. When clients are feeling stuck in their individual work, for example, I may encourage them to bring in their partner or family members to provide input and perspective. Exploring relational dynamics can be a powerful catalyst for change that can help not only the client but significant others in their lives as well. You may consider a change in treatment modality such as trying a group therapy approach rather than individual treatment. Or you may want to opt for a therapist who takes a different approach to counseling, for example, someone who focuses more on emotions if your previous therapist helped you examine your thought processes (you will read more about the different approaches to treatment in chaps. 2 and 4).

Please consider giving psychotherapy another try. When you do, tell your new counselor about your previous experience in therapy. It is highly likely that you and your therapist can develop a plan for a more beneficial therapy experience.

SEEKING COUNSELING AT THE ENCOURAGEMENT OF OTHERS

You may have been encouraged to enter counseling at the insistence of others, including family, friends, medical providers, and employers. Hearing the words from someone "Have you thought about seeing a counselor?" can potentially trigger defensiveness, resistance, and the self-assertion that "I'm fine!" However, it is worth considering whether your significant others can see areas of concern from their vantage point that you may not yet be able to see for yourself. Their expressions of concern convey their hope for you for a better life that you may not yet be able to envision.

If you have been encouraged to seek counseling but are not sure you see the need, it is to your benefit to give it a chance. Put your doubts, questions, and skepticism about psychotherapy out there in the first session. Give yourself the opportunity to discover whether there is something you can gain from the counseling experience.

Action Step: Self-Assessment of Mental Health

As we approach the end of the chapter, I encourage you to take a few minutes to reflect on the questions below and consider your mental health status. If the list feels too long, please choose the questions that are most relevant for you. This would be a great time to get out your journal and jot down some notes as you contemplate whether this is the right time to begin the counseling journey. Consider sharing your responses with a trusted mentor, friend, or family member.

Questions for Reflection

- Where do I hope for change in my life?
- How is my overall sense of mental and emotional well-being?
- How well am I able to cope with the stressors in my life?
- Am I able to recognize and use my capabilities in a meaningful way in my work, school, and volunteer activities?
- How would I describe the quality and satisfaction of my relationships with others?
- What are my risk factors for developing mental health symptoms (bio-psycho-social-spiritual)?
- What are the protective factors that I can draw from to improve my mental health and well-being?
- Have I sufficiently processed my experiences of suffering, grief, or trauma?
- What spiritual or existential questions do I continue to struggle with?
- Which of the barriers to accessing mental health treatment do I resonate with?
- Am I ready to ask for help and talk to someone about my problems?

Summing Up

We have come full circle to our original question: "Why should I consider psychotherapy?" I hope this chapter has provided the needed incentive to mind your mental health, improve your quality of life, strengthen spiritual vitality, and enhance your capacity to cope with inevitable life challenges. It is completely understandable to have some degree of apprehension about seeking psychotherapy and to feel challenged by the very real barriers that exist to accessing and affording mental health care. Your decision to read this book is an important first step to dispelling myths and demystifying the process so you can make an informed choice about how best to set out on your own journey toward enhanced mental health and well-being.

In her excellent TED talk "Why You Should Try Therapy Yesterday," Dr. Emily Anhalt describes psychotherapy as the life-changing experience of finding "a trained, objective person to help you understand your own mind."[23] When you have tried again and again to find solutions to the problems that plague you, you come to a point where you begin to lose hope that your life can ever change. By contemplating the counseling journey, you have taken a hopeful step toward the richer, fuller life that is available to you.

Roles Recap: Why Should I Consider Counseling?

THERAPIST ROLE	CLIENT ROLE
Respond to client inquiries about counseling and how it can help	Know the signs and symptoms of mental health issues
Help clients explore both risk and protective factors for mental health issues	Conduct an honest self-assessment of readiness and need for counseling
Make every effort to remove potential barriers to counseling to increase client access to services	Identify potential barriers to accessing counseling
Respond to client questions about financial arrangements for counseling and work with clients to increase access to services	Explore financial resources for counseling, including health insurance coverage
Provide accurate information about the costs and benefits of counseling so clients can make an informed choice	Make an informed choice about your readiness for counseling and share your decision with a trusted friend or mentor

---

[23]Emily Anhalt, "Why You Should Try Therapy Yesterday," TedXBoulder, October 19, 2019, 10:50, www.youtube.com/watch?v=eE6Rt-bFkvw.

2

Choosing a Therapist
as a Trustworthy Guide

*My physician referred me to you. I am having these episodes where
I have difficulty breathing, dizziness, my heart is pounding, and
I get a stomachache. I tried yoga and deep breathing to manage
my stress, but it hasn't helped. I have been calling in sick to work
more and more because I am afraid of having another episode. My
medical tests are all normal, and my doctor recommended I talk to
a psychologist to get help dealing with the stress in my life. I have
never seen a counselor before, and I am not sure how counseling
can help me; I feel nervous about telling my problems to a stranger.
But I am desperate to get some relief from these symptoms.*

PHONE CONVERSATION WITH A PROSPECTIVE CLIENT

The decision to start out on the counseling journey can feel a little
like deciding to climb Mount Everest: a risky and daunting under-
taking that you would not dare to take on alone. Like the client above,
you may know you need help but may be unfamiliar with the counseling process and unsure where to begin to find out about treatment
options. You need a sure-footed partner to show the way, share the
burden, and keep you on the path to health. Enter your own psychological guide—the therapist.

Once you have made the important decision to pursue psychotherapy,
the next part of the process involves choosing a mental health provider
to be a trustworthy guide for the counseling journey. In this chapter, I
will describe the treatment options and types of providers available,
answer some common questions about choosing a therapist, and get

down to the details about what kinds of questions to ask when talking to prospective therapists. The choices can be a bit overwhelming, but educating yourself about treatment options can be empowering, it can optimize the fit between you and your therapist, and it can instill confidence in the counseling experience.

Continuum of Treatment Options

An internet search of counseling services will usually result in a confusing array of treatment options, from self-help groups to residential treatment centers. While this book focuses on psychotherapy, it can be helpful to know that mental health treatment is available on a continuum of care. Clients and providers work together to assess the appropriate level of care by evaluating the severity and pervasiveness of symptoms. If you are experiencing mental health symptoms, it is essential to know that you have many options. Let's look briefly at the continuum of care available to clients.

Preventative care. Like our client in the quotation at the start of this chapter, people with mild symptoms of short duration may opt to try preventative strategies to address their distress or discomfort. Preventative care includes seeking social support, joining a support group, exercising, improving nutrition, and using mindfulness practices. If symptoms do not improve or worsen, seeing a mental health professional for assessment and treatment recommendations is an important next step.

Psychoeducation is a type of preventative care that involves in-person or online seminars, workshops, and support groups taught by mental health professionals or paraprofessionals that provide information about common challenges and coping strategies. Community organizations, churches, and professional groups offer in-person and online psychoeducation opportunities on topics such as relationship enrichment, grief support, parent training, and divorce recovery. Psychoeducation can help people identify common risk factors and learn preventative strategies to offset the development of more severe psychological symptoms.

Self-help groups provide peer support and counseling for addressing behavioral or psychological challenges. Groups offer the opportunity to come together with others who may be experiencing similar challenges for mutual support and help. Examples of self-help groups include Alcoholics Anonymous, Celebrate Recovery, and National Alliance on Mental Illness.

Many churches offer pastoral care as well as lay counseling programs, such as Stephen Ministries, which provides trained listeners to walk alongside people struggling with life challenges and mental health issues.[1] Lay counselors can provide needed support and help to determine when a referral to a professional is required.

If you are not sure whether you need to see a counselor or are on a waiting list for a provider, engaging in psychoeducation and self-help opportunities can provide valuable support and helpful resources.

Outpatient counseling and psychotherapy. As described in chapter one, counseling and psychotherapy involve the provision of psychological treatment to individuals, couples, and families in an office, clinic, or hospital setting. To help the client in the quotation at the beginning of this chapter, a mental health professional would meet with the client for an initial assessment, explore the history and severity of their symptoms, and then work with them to develop a treatment plan customized to their needs and goals. Outpatient therapy groups are also available and provide the added benefit for clients of learning from the experiences of others and normalizing their current struggles. Perhaps this anxious client would also benefit from a group for clients who struggle with panic disorder, for example. Holistic outpatient treatment of mental health issues may also involve a recommendation for complementary therapy, such as consultation with a dietitian, educational specialist, career counselor, or spiritual director.

Treatment programs. Day treatment, intensive outpatient, and partial hospitalization programs provide increasing levels of support for

---

[1] Information and training resources for Stephen Ministries can be found on their website, www.stephenministries.org/.

individuals requiring a more intensive level of intervention. Care coordination is provided by a multidisciplinary team led by a psychiatrist or psychologist. Treatment usually involves a combination of individual therapy, group counseling, psychoeducation, and psychiatric care. Faith-based treatment programs are available in some geographic areas. Suppose the client above is increasingly unable to function or engage in their job. In that case, they may benefit from an intensive treatment program for support in dealing with their debilitating anxiety symptoms.

Inpatient psychiatric hospitalization. Hospitalization may be required for clients who are at risk of harming themselves or others, need stabilization of acute psychological symptoms, or require detoxification related to substance abuse. Inpatient hospitalization provides short-term, 24-7 medical treatment and monitoring under the care of a psychiatrist. Treatment usually involves psychiatric evaluation, individual and group therapy, and complementary treatments such as expressive and occupational therapies. After stabilization of acute symptoms, patients are typically discharged to a partial hospitalization or day treatment program to continue treatment for additional days or weeks.

Residential treatment centers. Sometimes people need longer-term structured care as live-in residents for a variety of behavioral health issues, including substance abuse, eating disorders, psychological trauma, and chronic mental health conditions. Treatment focuses on stabilizing symptoms through therapeutic interventions delivered in a community context. Faith-based residential treatment centers are available that deliver professional care from a faith perspective.

Crisis intervention. There are times when emotional distress is so significant that immediate care is warranted. Crisis intervention services are necessary when acute psychological symptoms are present, as they provide immediate assessment and connection with the appropriate level of care. If you have active thoughts of harming yourself or harming another, please call the suicide and crisis lifeline by dialing 988 (if you are in the US), where you will be connected with a local crisis center that can provide confidential support twenty-four hours a day, seven days a week. Alternatively, you can visit your local hospital's emergency room to receive crisis assessment and intervention. If you are concerned that someone you know may be in immediate danger of harming themselves or others, or if they are having a psychiatric emergency, you can call 911 and ask for a wellness check on the person. Many countries around the world offer crisis assistance and you can find a list of crisis hotlines by country through Find a Helpline at www.iasp.info /crisis-centres-helplines.

If you are in doubt about what level of treatment is needed for your symptoms right now, you do not have to figure this out on your own. A medical or mental health professional can provide a confidential assessment to help you make this determination.

The Who's Who of Mental Health Professionals

There are many types of mental health professionals to choose from, and this section will provide a brief comparison to help you find the best fit for your counseling needs. Professionals who offer counseling and psychotherapy include psychiatrists, psychologists, counselors, marriage and family therapists, clinical social workers, and pastoral counselors. Mental health professionals may provide individual, couple, group, or family counseling. These professionals share a base of knowledge and common terminology but have different emphases in terms of specializations.

- Psychiatrists utilize a medical-model approach and can prescribe medication.
- Psychologists provide psychotherapy, consultation, and psychological evaluations using approaches and techniques based on the best existing research.
- Counselors provide guidance to help clients deal with challenges and meet their life goals.
- Marriage and family therapists specialize in family systems approaches, which often involve more than one person in the therapy room.

- Clinical social workers provide counseling services and may specialize in case management and advocacy for clients to access community resources.

- Pastoral counselors and chaplains provide counseling and spiritual guidance.

Each profession has a specific credentialing process, which includes education, supervised experience, and professional licensure (see table 2.1 for a comparison). Overall, the differences between individual therapists are most often more significant within the various disciplines than between, but it is helpful for the thoughtful consumer to know the differences. In the end, choosing a therapist you can connect with and trust will have a more significant impact on a positive therapy outcome than their specific degree or specialty.

THE IMPORTANCE OF THE PSYCHOTHERAPY RELATIONSHIP

The *psychotherapy relationship* or *therapeutic alliance* is the trust, connection, and collaboration that develops between the therapist and client during the counseling process. Over the past five decades, research has consistently demonstrated the importance of the therapy relationship for successful therapy outcomes.[a] A primary goal of the early stages of counseling is the development of trust and connection between the client and therapist, which then serves as a foundation for the counseling work. The therapeutic bond is developed as counselors demonstrate empathy, positive regard, genuineness, and respect toward clients by using a collaborative and flexible approach to therapy goals and interventions that respects client preferences, personality, and characteristics. The therapy relationship is strengthened as therapists seek out and respond to client feedback about the therapy experience and also seek to repair any relational ruptures that occur during the process.

[a]John C. Norcross and Michael J. Lambert, "Psychotherapy Relationships That Work III," *Psychotherapy* 55 (2018): 303-15, https://doi.org/10.1037/pst0000193.

The education and training process for mental health professionals includes at least two years of graduate education and one year of supervised experience for master's-level counselors, at least four years of graduate education plus two years of supervised experience for doctoral-level psychologists, and four years of medical school plus a four-year residency for psychiatrists. Licensure requirements vary state by state and include supervised experience plus completion of licensure examinations. If you are pursuing services through a community mental health center or university training clinic, you may be assigned to a therapist-in-training, which is often the most cost-effective option. While it is true that they will have less experience than a fully licensed professional, therapists-in-training are closely supervised by credentialed professionals, and clients can benefit from having more than one professional involved in their treatment.

During our formal education and throughout our careers, most psychotherapists engage in our own personal therapy to deepen our understanding of "person-of-the-therapist" issues and to deal with our own problems and challenges. Mental health professionals are somewhat unique among healthcare providers in that the self of the therapist is one of the most significant resources we bring to the treatment process. It is immensely helpful for us to experience the other side of the couch so we can be the best possible therapist for our clients. My own experiences as a client have been instrumental in forming who I am as a clinician and have inspired me to re-create the high level of therapeutic trust and partnership that were so beneficial to me as I navigated my own mental health journey.

How Important Is Finding a Therapist with Expertise in Your Specific Issues?

Licensed mental health professionals are trained to work effectively with a wide range of presenting problems. However, most therapists also have areas of specialization where they have received advanced training, credentials, and supervised experience. Therapists will usually list their areas of expertise in their online bio, or you can ask about their knowledge and expertise during a phone call to explore goodness of fit. A good rule of thumb is that the more pervasive, severe, and debilitating your condition, the more helpful it will be to find a therapist who specializes in treating your symptoms. The following is a brief review of some common mental health issues people bring to counseling, with special considerations for choosing a therapist.

Depression and anxiety symptoms. As I discussed in chapter one, the number of individuals struggling with symptoms of depression and anxiety has increased significantly following the pandemic, and it is one of the most common reasons people seek out counseling and psychotherapy. There are many types of depression and anxiety disorders on the spectrum of symptoms that occur in response to stressful life events (called adjustment disorders) to more severe and debilitating mood and anxiety disorders, including bipolar disorders, major depressive disorders, panic disorders, and obsessive-compulsive disorders.

Nearly all licensed mental health providers are qualified to provide assessment and treatment of depression and anxiety symptoms. However, clients suffering from severe and debilitating symptoms will want to make sure they choose a therapist with expertise in the treatment of their depression and anxiety symptoms and may also benefit from evaluation by a psychiatrist for medication.

Trauma-related symptoms and posttraumatic stress disorder. Most of us will experience a traumatic event at some point during our lives. The American Psychological Association provides this definition: "Trauma involves events that pose a significant threat (physical, emotional, or psychological) to the safety of the victim or loved ones/friends and are overwhelming and shocking."[2] Witnessing or experiencing a traumatic event often results in distressing symptoms, including disturbing memories or flashbacks of the trauma, avoidance of situations or stimuli related to the trauma, distressing emotions and thoughts, and higher-than-normal levels of reactivity. For most people, these distressing symptoms fade away on their own. However, for some, the effects can linger and be quite debilitating.

---

[2]"Clinical Practice Guideline for the Treatment of Post Traumatic Stress Disorder (PTSD) in Adults," American Psychological Association, February 24, 2017: ES-3, www.apa.org /ptsd-guideline/ptsd.pdf.

Trauma-informed care refers to treatment approaches that prioritize the provision of a safe and trustworthy environment for healing to occur. Effective trauma-informed treatments help clients gradually process the thoughts, emotions, memories, and physical symptoms that have continued after the traumatic event. Trauma-informed care also teaches clients coping skills for dealing with the disruptive thoughts, feelings, and physiological symptoms that can occur when reprocessing the trauma. Through effective treatment, distressing symptoms decrease, and clients can find relief from trauma-related symptoms.

If you are struggling with symptoms related to a traumatic event, whether recent or in the distant past, trauma-informed therapy can be highly beneficial. For some clients, the desire to avoid thinking about and remembering difficult events can be a barrier to seeking out the very treatment that can alleviate their distress. However, effective treatments are available, and finding a therapist with expertise in trauma treatment is an important first step on the pathway to hope and healing.

Special consideration in the treatment of addictions. Addictions affect a significant number of adolescents and adults worldwide and can include drugs, alcohol, tobacco, gambling, pornography, and compulsive overeating. A 2021 Substance Abuse and Mental Health Services Administration survey found that substance use disorders were highest among eighteen to twenty-five year old young adults (26 percent), followed by adults (16 percent) and adolescents (8.5 percent).[3] Anyone who has attempted to overcome an addiction on their own knows the shame and helplessness that can result in the vicious cycle of recovery and relapse. While some individuals can successfully overcome addiction independently, most benefit significantly from a combination of support groups (such as twelve-step programs) and psychotherapy targeting the thoughts, emotions, and behaviors that maintain the addiction.

When looking for addiction treatment, start with an online search of support groups in your area, such as Alcoholics Anonymous, Gamblers

---

[3]"National Survey of Drug Use and Health (NSDUH) Releases, 2021," Substance Abuse and Mental Health Services Administration, 2021, 36, www.samhsa.gov/data/release /2021-national-survey-drug-use-and-health-nsduh-releases.

Anonymous, or Overeaters Anonymous. The more severe the addiction, the more critical it is to find a therapist with specialized training in the treatment of addiction as indicated by a specialty certification. Inquire with prospective therapists about their experience and approach in the treatment of addictions. Ask sponsors and members of your twelve-step group for recommendations of good addiction specialists. If you are struggling with both an addiction and a mental health condition at the same time, finding a therapist who specializes in co-occurring substance use and mental disorders will be necessary. For a faith-based approach to addiction treatment, consider a twelve-step program based on Christian principles such as Celebrate Recovery, with online and in-person meetings across the United States.[4]

When family, couple, or relational problems are the main issue. Increasingly, people seek professional help to treat problems in their primary relationships. Couple and family therapists can provide expertise in assessing and treating common relational difficulties, including communication, parent-child problems, conflict resolution, sexual intimacy issues, and infidelity. Engaging in couple or family therapy proactively before problems begin, with premarital counseling for example, can help build a foundation of relational trust, communication, and problem solving that can prevent the development of future relational problems. If you identify issues in relationships as the primary reason for wanting to pursue counseling, consider seeking out a provider with a specialization in couple or family therapy, such as a licensed marriage and family therapist who can provide a systemic approach to counseling that treats the relationship as the primary client.

Sometimes, only one partner or family member is willing to come to counseling to address the current relationship problems. While you cannot change other people, you can change your part in interactional patterns in your relationships and thus affect the entire couple or family system. Plus, individual counseling for relationship issues can provide

---

[4]For information on how to find a Celebrate Recovery group, see https://celebraterecovery .com.

a place for support and problem solving for clients experiencing inter-personal challenges.

Finding a therapist for your child or adolescent. As a parent or care-giver, you may be looking for a competent mental health professional to help with problems related to your child or adolescent, and I can offer you this practical advice. It is important to find someone with specialized training and experience in the assessment and treatment of childhood mental health issues who will recognize the common developmental needs and challenges that children experience. You will also want someone who can connect well with your child and also with you as a parent. For most child and adolescent concerns, family therapy and/or parent coaching and support are integral to treatment. Child treatment often involves games, art, activities, and other age-appropriate alternatives to talk therapy.

The older your child is, the more you will want them to have input regarding the choice of a therapist. I advise parents to do the initial screening of therapists online or by phone, narrowing down a list of providers who meet parents' criteria for professional qualifications and affordability. Then, share what you have learned with your adolescent and ask for their input. Schedule an initial appointment with the agreed-upon therapist for both you and your child to ensure goodness of fit.

It is vital to clarify confidentiality practices, which vary by state, when your child is seeing a mental health provider. Generally, parents have access to their minor child's medical records but also want to respect the privacy of their child's counseling sessions to build trust between the child and therapist. My own practice is to provide parents with regular updates on treatment, most often in the presence of their child to maintain trust.

When should I consider medication? A common question for many clients is whether medication will alleviate their psychological symptoms. As discussed earlier in the chapter, psychotherapists do not prescribe medication (except some states where psychologists have prescription privileges), but we can help clients determine whether a consultation with a psychiatrist would be a beneficial part of their treatment plan. If a referral to a psychiatrist is made, the therapists and psychiatrist will likely work together to monitor the client's progress and determine the best course of treatment. A psychiatric consultation involves evaluation by a physician to determine whether medication is an option for treating mental health symptoms. Clients are seen for an initial evaluation and then monitored through follow-up visits.

We know that some mental health conditions have significant biologically based etiology and will likely respond best to medication to alleviate symptoms, for example, bipolar disorders and psychotic disorders.[5] For some depressive disorders, a combination of psychotherapy and medication may yield the best treatment outcomes. For other types of disorders, including anxiety, addictions, and relational and family issues, psychotherapy is usually the most effective approach. However, medication can provide some relief from debilitating symptoms related to these conditions.

What About Telehealth Therapy Options? Are They Effective?

Telepsychology, or the provision of psychological services through electronic platforms (phone, video conference, email, texting, etc.), has been around for a number of years but has grown tremendously in availability and popularity since the Covid-19 pandemic. Counseling services transitioned literally overnight from in-person office visits to online platforms. Many therapists and clients have found benefits in the convenience and ease of access provided by telemental health care. What do we know about the effectiveness of psychotherapy delivered online?

Research on the effectiveness of telemental health care has found that generally, most clients receive benefits equivalent to those of in-person therapy in terms of the reduction of symptoms. These research outcomes have been demonstrated for a variety of mental health conditions, including severe mental illness and substance use disorders.[6]

---

[5]For a good overview of evidence-based treatment approaches including psychological conditions that benefit from medication as part of the treatment plan, see APA Division 12 (Society of Clinical Psychology), "How Do I Choose Between Medication and Psychotherapy?," American Psychological Association, www.apa.org/ptsd-guideline/patients -and-families/medication-or-therapy.
[6]Substance Abuse and Mental Health Services Administration, "Telehealth for the Treatment of Serious Mental Illness and Substance Use Disorders," SAMHSA publication no. PEP21-06-02-001, 2021, www.govinfo.gov/content/pkg/GOVPUB-HE20-PURL -gpo156347/pdf/GOVPUB-HE20-PURL-gpo156347.pdf.

Additionally, clients with limited mobility or transportation diffi-culties may find teletherapy an excellent option. Clients who are con-cerned about the stigma of seeing a therapist may find online therapy less anxiety-producing than walking into a therapist's office. Essential elements for a good teletherapy experience include having a private place for sessions, access and ability to use technology, and reliable internet service.

However, telepsychology may not be the best treatment for ev-eryone. In addition to personal preference, some clients may find it harder to connect with a therapist online or discover they are more easily distracted during remote sessions. Others find it challenging to locate a private space to hold their online sessions. During the pan-demic, I conducted many sessions with clients who resorted to sitting in their vehicle in the driveway for privacy, which was very chal-lenging during our chilly Chicago winters! Research on the impact of teletherapy on the psychotherapy relationship shows mixed results; some studies show no difference, while in other studies, both clients and therapists rate the therapeutic alliance lower during online therapy. Some types of therapy that are enhanced by physical presence, such as exposure therapy for anxiety, or role-playing, may be more difficult to deliver online. Clients may also prefer to have the in-person presence of a therapist when dealing with difficult feelings and experiences. Clients with high distractibility, sensory difficulties, or limited comfort and literacy with technology may not be suitable for teletherapy.[7]

Online services have proliferated that provide easy access to a tele-health therapist for a self-pay subscription fee.[8] These services usually require clients to complete a brief assessment and then provide a match with a therapist, charging a monthly subscription fee. Online services have made therapy more accessible for many who do not want

---

[7]Rebecca Appleton et al., "Implementation, Adoption, and Perceptions of Telemental Health During the COVID-19 Pandemic: Systematic Review," Journal of Medical Internet Research 23 (2021), doi:10.2196/31746.

[8]See, for example, Better Help, www.betterhelp.com, or Talkspace, www.talkspace.com.

the hassle of trying to find a therapist on their own. However, many people prefer to be able to choose their own therapist and ensure that they are appropriately credentialed with professional licensure and experience. In addition, it is often financially advantageous for clients to opt for telehealth services covered by their health insurance, which may be more cost-efficient than a monthly self-pay subscription to an online service.

My own experience of telepsychology over the past few years has been mixed. I have been pleasantly surprised by the effectiveness of individual, couple, and family therapy conducted online, mostly with clients with whom I had already established a solid therapy relationship but also with some clients I have never met in person. Many of my clients prefer in-person sessions as our regular practice whenever possible, and we use telehealth sessions periodically. For me, there is something essential and intangible about being physically present with clients in the same room that adds depth and substance to our work together. God created us with human bodies, and in the process of healing, the incarnational aspects of presence can be invaluable for growth and transformation.

Faith Perspectives: How Important Is It for Me to See a Christian Counselor?

For many religious clients, choosing a therapist who respects and understands their religious values and commitments is a priority. Integrating religious and spiritual practices into the counseling experience leads to positive outcomes for Christian clients, as evidenced by improvements in both mental health and spiritual well-being.[9] I believe that when I help clients move toward human flourishing, they are also moving closer to God's desire and intent for their lives. As therapists, we want our clients to bring all aspects of themselves to the counseling journey toward health and wholeness of body, mind, and soul.

---

[9]Everett L. Worthington, "Research on the Efficacy of Christian Counseling," *Christian Counseling Today* 24, no. 1 (2021), www.aacc.net/2021/01/29/research-on-the-efficacy-of -christian-counseling/.

As a psychologist and professor of psychology, it has been a great joy to teach at an educational institution that encourages the integration of Christian faith and practice with psychology, counseling, and family therapy. We have the opportunity to educate and mentor students who have dedicated their careers to serving church and society with their counseling skills. If it is important to you to see a counselor who shares your faith commitments, be encouraged to know that there are many exceptional Christian clinicians around the world who can provide counseling expertise from a Christian worldview to help you integrate your spiritual and psychological journeys.

"How do I find a Christian therapist?" is a question I frequently hear from friends and colleagues. Clients searching for a Christian therapist may encounter a confusing array of professional titles and descriptions. In this section, we will consider some types of Christian counselors, differences in their training and education, and guidelines for determining which option might be the best for you.

Christian mental health professionals. This group of professionals includes licensed psychologists, counselors, clinical social workers, marriage and family therapists, and psychiatrists who integrate their Christian faith with professional best practices. Professionals in this category have completed a graduate degree in a mental health field, including supervised clinical practice, before obtaining professional licensure from their respective states. Their professional services are covered by health insurance and governed by their respective disciplines' ethical codes of conduct. They may or may not explicitly advertise their services as Christian counseling, as some provide services for clients from diverse religious backgrounds.

Professionals in this category may differ in how explicitly they integrate their Christian faith with counseling, psychology, and family therapy principles. They will have diverse educational backgrounds, with some receiving education at faith-based graduate schools, while others may have graduated from secular institutions. Generally, Christian mental health professionals integrate Christian theology, biblical wisdom, and spiritual practices with psychological theory, research, and interventions.

Pastoral counselors and chaplains. These professionals are often dual credentialed with education and training in counseling techniques, Christian theology, and ministry. They may be ordained in their denomination and provide counseling services through a church, hospital, military, or community-based organization. Pastoral counselors and chaplains may or may not be licensed by their respective states. Chaplain services may be covered by health insurance, mostly when they occur in a hospital setting. Many chaplains and pastoral counselors focus primarily on spiritual guidance and soul care while integrating counseling principles and practices.

Biblical counselors. These counselors view Scripture as the primary source of wisdom and guidance for counseling and may or may not draw on principles or interventions from professional counseling and psychology. Although biblical counselors are not formally licensed by the state in which they practice, many have completed training and certification programs and hold specific credentials, abiding by their credentialing program's ethical guidelines.[10] Biblical counselors focus on ministering to others by offering biblical guidance.

Spiritual directors. Spiritual directors are found in many denominations and focus on guiding individuals in their spiritual journey. Most spiritual directors receive specialized mentoring or training in the practice of spiritual direction and provide their services through churches, retreat centers, and ministries. Individuals seek spiritual direction to aid their spiritual growth, strengthen their relationship with God, deepen their prayer life, or for spiritual discernment and growth.

Factors to consider. Counseling and psychotherapy are different from other types of health care in that psychotherapy often triggers spiritual questions, just as spiritual issues can have a psychological impact. Even though all therapists are ethically bound to work within the client's value system and not impose their own, seeing a counselor

---

[10]For a definition of biblical counseling and information about the certification process, see Association of Certified Biblical Counselors, https://biblicalcounseling.com/.

who shares a client's own religious commitments may be optimal for building a foundation of trust and confidence in the process. However, it may not always be possible or expedient to find a Christian therapist, particularly if you are in the midst of a mental health crisis and need immediate care. Your provider choices may be limited due to your geographic area or insurance policy. Let us use the following hypothetical case example to highlight important considerations.

Isaac is in his first year of college and has been experiencing extreme mood swings that interfere with his academic and social activities. On some days, he is too depressed to get out of bed to attend class. On other days, he feels confident and energetic but struggles with racing thoughts and difficulties focusing. It is clear that he needs assessment and treatment by a mental health professional. How important is it that Isaac see a Christian counselor?

Due to the severity and debilitating nature of Isaac's symptoms, he needs to seek treatment as soon as possible for an accurate diagnosis and intervention. Given the nature of his symptoms, it is likely he will require an evaluation by a psychiatrist to consider medication that may help stabilize his symptoms so he can participate in school. For Isaac, professional expertise and speedy access will be primary considerations when choosing a therapist.

Let's say that Isaac, as a committed Christian, has also found that spiritual practices such as contemplative prayer and Scripture study have helped him navigate the difficulties of his mood swings. He wants to make sure that he sees a therapist who understands and respects his spiritual practices and can help him improve both his mental health and his relationship with God. He has questions about why God has not healed him from these symptoms, and these religious doubts contribute to his depressive symptoms. Given the importance of Isaac's religious coping as well as his spiritually distressing questions, he would benefit from seeing a Christian mental health professional who can integrate his mental health treatment with his faith journey.

To continue the scenario, let us imagine that Isaac has connected with a Christian therapist and a psychiatrist. He is now taking medication to help stabilize his mood swings and is learning coping skills in therapy for regulating his emotions, strengthening his social support, and meeting his academic challenges. However, he continues to be plagued by spiritual questions and doubts, which were precipitated by the loss of a beloved grandparent shortly before Isaac left for college. He is struggling with questions about life after death and is unsure of his salvation. While it will be beneficial for Isaac to talk about these issues in therapy to explore the psychological aspects of his spiritual concerns, he would also benefit from meeting with a pastoral counselor, spiritual director, or spiritual mentor who can provide biblical and theological guidance and ongoing discipleship.

It can be challenging to know what we need when we are in the midst of suffering and whether our issues are primarily psychological, spiritual, or both (which is usually the case!). Bottom line: do not delay treatment if you are in acute distress and finding it difficult to function in your daily life. It is essential to start somewhere in your journey toward mental and spiritual health, and you can always change directions along the way or add other helping professionals to your support network.

Ultimately, clients have the right to choose the therapist that is the best fit for them, and it is perfectly acceptable to inquire about a prospective therapist's religious orientation before deciding on a counselor. I recommend asking some key questions to help determine whether the fit is likely to be successful, including the following:

- What is your professional background—education, training, licensure, credentials?
- What professional ethical code do you adhere to?
- How do you incorporate Christian beliefs and practices into your counseling services?
- Are your services covered by health insurance?

If you are unable to access a Christian provider, do not lose hope. Our ethical codes bind all mental health professionals to respect our clients' diverse backgrounds and values, including religious commitments. As a practicing psychologist, I am dedicated to providing respectful, inclusive, and competent psychotherapy for all of my clients, regardless of their religious identity or background. Talk with your therapist about your desire to incorporate your faith into your counseling experience and actively draw from spiritual resources during your treatment. If you feel dissatisfied by the way religious and spiritual issues are being addressed, raise these concerns with your therapist.

Action Step: Specific Strategies for Finding a Therapist

Choosing the right therapist is an important first step in the counseling journey, and it is worth investing the extra time and energy in finding someone you can connect well with. You will want to look for a credentialed, licensed therapist who has experience with your presenting problems. Because of the importance of the psychotherapy relationship for successful treatment outcomes, look for a therapist who is committed to understanding your problems within your personal context. For this reason, some clients may have preferences about the therapist's characteristics, such as gender, race, ethnicity, or religious affiliation. Table 2.2 provides some websites that can help get you started in finding a therapist.

The first step in choosing a counselor is to research your insurance coverage for behavioral health or mental health services. Find out from your insurance company whether a referral from your primary care physician is needed to initiate services and whether there is a list of providers you will need to choose from. Inquire about the different reimbursement rates for in-network and out-of-network providers. Ask a trusted friend or professional to review your list of in-network providers to highlight the names of therapists that they would recommend.

For a more targeted therapist search, ask for recommendations from trusted professionals such as primary care physicians, religious leaders, and professional colleagues. Employers or schools may have referral lists of preferred therapists. Your human resources department can also point you in the right direction, and may recommend that you begin utilizing services through an employee assistance program. Another option is to use online therapist directories that support therapist

searches by credentials, location, specialization, and therapist characteristics. Many organizations will also have a list of therapists special-
izing in a specific type of mental health concern or problem.

If finances are a barrier to accessing mental health care, good options for finding a therapist include community mental health centers,
university-based training clinics, or requesting a reduced or sliding-
scale fee from prospective providers. Don't give up! If you run out of
options, you can enlist friends and family members to help in your search.

Once you have your list of top choices, you can initiate contact by
phone for a brief conversation to determine the therapist's goodness of
fit and availability. After briefly sharing why you are interested in therapy,
consider asking the following questions:

- Are you accepting new clients?
- What is your experience with my type of problem?
- Do you have a particular approach to therapy that you use?
- What is your experience working with clients from my cultural/
  religious background?
- What are your fees and insurance billing practices?

You will likely need to speak with several therapists before finding the
best fit, and I encourage you not to get discouraged if this takes a couple
of weeks. Some clients may find it more convenient to schedule the first
session through email or online office portals, and then questions can
be explored during the initial session. Once contact is made and the
appointment with the counselor is set, many clients experience a
glimmer of hope and positive expectation for change, which can lead to
symptom improvement even before the first session. While this is encouraging, following through with the appointment is important to
ensure that improvements and positive changes are sustained.

One of my clients encouraged me to pass along this sensible advice
for choosing a therapist: "When I talked to therapists on the phone, I
just had a gut feeling about who I would connect with best, and I was
right! Don't be afraid to tell a prospective therapist that you do not feel

we would be a good fit to work together. Hold out for the one that feels right. Trust your gut!"

Summing Up

This chapter provides an overview of treatment options, types of providers, and common questions for clients when choosing a trustworthy guide for the counseling journey. As a next step, I encourage you to develop a short list of two to four therapists from your search. Make a commitment to call each one and test the waters to see whether there is a good connection. Sometimes it can take several phone calls or emails to find the right person with an opening for new clients. Try to keep your search going even if this takes some time. When you find the right fit, make a choice and schedule that first appointment. Congratulations—your counseling journey has begun!

Roles Recap: Finding a Therapist

THERAPIST ROLES	CLIENT ROLES
Complete educational, professional, and licensure requirements to provide counseling and psychotherapy services to the public	Research financial resources for therapy through your employer, insurance company, and community-based services
Pursue ongoing professional development of clinical expertise through continuing education	Gather names of referrals from health providers, community leaders, employers, and friends
Respond to new-client inquiries in a timely manner	Consider therapist characteristics that are important for building a strong therapy relationship
Answer prospective client questions about therapist credentials, experience, approach to counseling	Initiate contact and request information to determine the goodness of fit—and trust your gut!
Provide information about professional fees, insurance, and billing practices	Be persistent and keep going even if it is challenging to find someone who is the right fit *and* has openings for new clients
Provide a good-faith estimate of the cost of therapy for self-pay clients	Decide on a therapist and schedule an initial appointment

Table 2.1. Comparison of mental health professionals

	EDUCATION	LICENSURE	EXPERTISE
Psychiatrists	Doctor of medicine (MD) or doctor of osteopathic medicine (DO) with specialized psychiatric training	Licensed as physicians or medical doctors	Diagnosis and treatment; prescribe and monitor medication
Psychologists	Doctoral degree in psychology (PsyD) or philosophy (PhD) in psychology or a related field	Licensed as psychologists or clinical psychologists	Assessment, diagnosis, and treatment of mental health issues; research, prevention, education
Counselors	Master's degree in counseling, psychology, or a related field	Licensed as professional counselors or clinical mental health counselors	Evaluation and treatment of mental health issues; also expertise in career counseling and wellness-oriented counseling
Marriage and Family Therapists	Master's degree in marriage and family therapy or counseling with a marriage and family therapy specialization	Licensed as marriage and family therapists or counselors	Couple and family treatment
Clinical Social Workers	Master's degree in social work	Licensed clinical social worker	Evaluation and treatment of mental health issues; also expertise in case management and advocacy
Drug or Alcohol Counselors	Bachelor's or master's degree plus specialized training in substance abuse	Licensure or certification as a clinical alcohol or substance abuse counselor	Evaluation and treatment of problems with substance use, dependence, and addiction

	EDUCATION	LICENSURE	EXPERTISE
Chaplains or pastoral counselors	Clinical pastoral education (CPE)	Certification and/ or ordination	Faith-based guidance and support and counseling in church, community, or the workplace

Note: Others who may be involved in mental health care include primary care physicians, psychiatric nurses, and specialized therapists (art therapy, equine therapy, applied behavioral analysis, etc.).[11]

Table 2.2. Therapist finders and directories

(See www.ivpress.com/the-client-s-guide-to-therapy for the most updated list.)

ORGANIZATION	WEBSITE
Alcoholics Anonymous	www.aa.org/
American Association of Christian Counselors	https://connect.aacc.net/?search _type=distance
American Association of Marriage and Family Therapy	https://aamft.org/Directories/Find_a _Therapist.aspx
American Psychological Association	https://locator.apa.org/
Anxiety and Depression Association of America	https://members.adaa.org/search /custom.asp?id=4685
Black Mental Health Association	https://blackmentalhealth.com /connect-with-a-therapist/
Christian Asian Mental Health	https://camh.network/counselors/
Christian Association for Psychological Studies	https://caps.net/online-directory/
Inclusive Therapists	www.inclusivetherapists.com/
National Center for PTSD	www.ptsd.va.gov/gethelp/find _therapist.asp
SAMSHA—substance abuse and mental health services	https://findtreatment.gov/

---

[11]For additional information on mental health providers, see National Alliance on Mental Illness, "Types of Mental Health Professionals," updated April 2020, www.nami.org /About-Mental-Illness/Treatments/Types-of-Mental-Health-Professionals/.

3

Beginning Well
and the Importance of
the Therapy Relationship

Client: Who is this person? Can I trust them? Will they
understand me? Will they judge me? Can they help me?

Therapist: How can I connect with this person?
What is their story? Where are they hurting?

CLIENT AND THERAPIST'S THOUGHTS
DURING A FIRST COUNSELING SESSION

Beginning well in therapy requires the development of trust and confidence in your therapist as a reliable guide for the counseling journey. Clients need to know that their counselor sees the way forward on the pathway to mental health, will help them carry their burdens, and ultimately enable them to reach their end goals. If *hope* propels you to undertake the counseling journey, then *trust* is the essential task of the initial phase of therapy.

Trust is essential to the formation of the therapeutic alliance, which is the emotional bond and working relationship between you and your therapist. Counseling and psychotherapy are unique among the health professions in that the professional relationship is especially central to the healing process and provides the space where important work occurs. Establishing a genuine human relationship is critical to this process, where both parties can bring their authentic selves to the encounter.

Understandably, many clients are apprehensive about telling their problems and concerns to someone they have just met. To help foster client comfort and safety, therapists offer interest, curiosity, empathy, respect, and confidentiality. Clients can then share their current struggles and problems honestly and often with great relief. A strong therapy relationship takes time to develop as you and your therapist figure out the best way to work together. Relationship ruptures and disruptions are inevitable, and addressing them through honest feedback and relational repair will only strengthen the trust and connection between you.

One aspect that sets counseling apart from other professions is that it is both *professional* and *personal*, in that the *person* of the therapist is essential to developing the strong psychotherapy relationship necessary for effective treatment to occur. Often, the authentically human aspects of the relationship create the conditions for successful outcomes in therapy, as we will see from a brief review of the science of psychotherapy. While it can be challenging to imagine sharing your personal struggles with another, it often does not take long to feel understood, supported, and hopeful about the potential for change.

Because of the importance of the relational aspects of the healing process, counselors spend quite a bit of time working on our own emotional and psychological health (and dealing with our own psychological baggage). This person-of-the-therapist work is an essential aspect of most educational and training programs, as we learn firsthand what is needed to work effectively on our own problems and challenges. As therapists, we are taking you on a healing journey that we ourselves have benefited from and will continue to make use of throughout our careers.

How do we begin the counseling journey and develop trust in the counselor and the psychotherapy process? Let's look at what to expect from the initial phase of the therapy process.

A Bird's-Eye View of the Counseling Experience

What does the counseling experience entail, and how does the process help clients along this journey toward mental health, well-being, and resilience? Many people expect psychotherapy to resemble the depictions of counseling portrayed in the media, some of which can be downright scary. No wonder we are apprehensive about the psychotherapy experience.

Instead of your worst therapy nightmare, imagine yourself meeting with a trusted professional who is both a guide and a fellow sojourner with you on the journey toward mental health. This reliable guide patiently helps you name and describe the problems, symptoms, and issues you have tried to deal with on your own without success. Picture this trusted and supportive guide bringing science-informed theory and practices to give you a new understanding of old problems. Together, you develop a treatment plan that respects your important cultural worldview and values. Rather than a passive patient undergoing a medical procedure, you, as a client, play an active role in your treatment, providing feedback about what works and what does not. As you share your burdens with another person who credibly bears witness to your life, you experience less shame and more hope. You recognize the strengths you have that you can draw from on the pathway to health and healing and discover other fellow travelers who can support you on the way.

All of us have experienced the healing power of social relationships. Sharing our problems and concerns with a skilled listener can bring a sense of relief, support, and normalization of our struggles. Throughout human history, body and soul care has occurred in the context of social relationships, where medical caregivers, community leaders, teachers, and spiritual advisers have brought competency and caring to heal the sick and wounded. There is something inherently curative about sharing emotional burdens with a trusted other who can listen empathically and nonjudgmentally and serve as an objective guide toward healing and health. Imagine the benefits of these social relationships supercharged with psychological knowledge and evidence-based strategies to bring about change. The benefits of these transformative conversations occurring in a *professional* relationship include confidentiality, client-centeredness, and skilled objectivity that is not present in other supportive social contexts.

While I will describe the counseling process in greater detail in the following chapters, it typically involves an initial assessment of the presenting problem, followed by collaborative goal setting and the development of a treatment plan with the general goal of reducing symptoms and facilitating personal growth. The therapist and client work together to determine the specific therapeutic approach to be used and to evaluate the effectiveness of the interventions, making necessary adjustments along the way. As therapeutic goals are met, clients decide together with their therapist when it is time to end therapy, with an open door to return if needed. Length of treatment can range from just a few sessions to longer-term services spanning several years, depending on the presenting problem, diagnosis, and treatment goals.

The client's own cultural and worldview commitments are highly relevant to the psychotherapy process as treatment approaches are adapted to each person's needs and values. All therapists have an ethical responsibility to respect client diversity, including age, gender, race and ethnicity, religion, national origin, sexual identity and orientation, socioeconomic status, and differential abilities, as part of our fundamental commitment to respect the dignity and worth of all human beings. For many clients, this includes consideration of their religious and spiritual commitments throughout the process of psychotherapy. When I meet with clients, I ask about what aspects of their background are important for us to include in the counseling process, and I make sure to incorporate this into our work together.

Developing Confidence in the Science Behind the Process

When considering an investment of time and money in psychotherapy, the thoughtful consumer must ask: "Does psychotherapy really work?" I have rarely had a client enter therapy and demand, "Show me the data!" However, few of us would undertake an important journey without doing a little research beforehand. Knowing some key findings from research on psychotherapy effectiveness can empower clients and therapists to trust the therapeutic journey confidently. Here are three takeaways from the research that can provide confidence and trust in the process and outcome of therapy.

First, hundreds of studies have been conducted that demonstrate that psychotherapy is highly beneficial for the treatment of a wide variety of mental health diagnoses.[1] Most people who undergo psychotherapy will experience positive change and a significant reduction of symptoms. This level of effectiveness is comparable to or better than treating psychological symptoms with psychiatric medication alone. Other good news is that the positive changes people gain from psychotherapy are maintained over time, even after treatment is concluded.[2]

Second, in addition to psychological benefits, psychotherapy contributes to better overall physical health, including a decrease in illness and greater longevity. Psychotherapy can reduce or prevent the onset of mental illness–related disability and result in better workplace functioning. It has also been demonstrated that counseling is efficacious in improving couple and family relationships, which significantly contributes to overall mental health. For many clients, the advantages of psychotherapy extend beyond the treatment of psychological symptoms and include personal growth and character change, making meaning of suffering, and emerging with a greater sense of purpose and direction.[3]

Third, we have learned quite a bit from scientific studies about how psychotherapy works. The effectiveness of psychotherapy is affected by several factors, including the client's personality characteristics and motivation, the therapist's characteristics, and most importantly, the strength and quality of the therapeutic working alliance.[4] It is critically important that clients trust their therapist and experience the necessary empathy, support, and respect so that problems and concerns can be

[1]Michael J. Lambert, "The Efficacy and Effectiveness of Psychotherapy," in *Bergin and Garfield's Handbook of Psychotherapy and Behavior Change*, 6th ed., ed. Michael Lambert (Hoboken, NJ: Wiley, 2012), 176.

[2]American Psychological Association, "Recognition of Psychotherapy Effectiveness," *Psychotherapy* 50, no. 1 (2013): 103, doi:10.1037/a0030276.

[3]American Psychological Association, "Recognition of Psychotherapy Effectiveness."

[4]Bruce Wampold and Zac E. Imel, *The Great Psychotherapy Debate*, 2nd ed. (New York: Routledge, 2015), 179-80.

shared honestly and openly. As therapists, we need to empathize with clients' concerns and provide treatment in a way that respects our client's culture and context. Ultimately, the client and therapist need to agree on their definition of the problem and the specific goals for treatment. This shared understanding gives the client hope and a positive expectancy for therapy, and this hope is a significant predictor of positive therapy outcomes.[5]

It is important to keep in mind that the specific approaches to therapy or techniques used by therapists are often less important than the strength of the therapeutic relationship for the effective treatment of most presenting problems.[6] One of the implications of this research finding is the importance of choosing a therapist based on the potential for a good relational connection, even more so than the therapist's specific theoretical approach or orientation.

The bottom line is that we can trust that psychotherapy effectively treats a wide variety of mental health issues and also fosters overall improvements in clients' health, functioning in the workplace, and relationships.

Can I Trust You? Establishing Trust as the Essential First Step

The starting place for all relationships, including the connection between clients and therapists, is the fundamental question, "Can I trust you?" The counseling journey starts with establishing a relationship of mutual trust that both parties can rely on throughout the process of therapy, especially when navigating the terrain becomes rocky.

For decades, scientists have been actively researching trust as an essential human need that is foundational for healthy relationships. Contemporary attachment theories suggest that our capacities for trust develop at an early age through those first relationships with caregivers, which then serve as a template for future relationships. Optimal relational capacities, or secure attachment, are developed when caregivers can provide a secure base for a child through responsiveness, attentiveness,

---

[5]Wampold and Imel, *Great Psychotherapy Debate*, 194-212.
[6]Wampold and Imel, *Great Psychotherapy Debate*, 156.

and consistency in responding to the child's needs. We carry the impact of these early relationships into adulthood as we seek trustworthy relationships throughout our lives.

Therapists draw from this developmental understanding of attachment theory as we seek to offer our clients a secure base in the counseling relationship through responsiveness, attentiveness, and consistency from the very first session through the end of the therapy experience. As clients feel safe, they can better engage in therapy and tolerate the painful emotional experiences that often occur as difficult memories and experiences are processed. This trust takes time to develop and has its ups, downs, and times of disconnection that require repair (more about this in chap. 6). It is common for clients to want to test the line and make sure their therapist is trustworthy before taking risks and climbing higher in their personal growth journey.

We can anticipate that the same challenges we encounter in our personal relationships will show up in the therapeutic relationship. I remember in my own therapy the moment when I recognized I was still trying to solve my problems independently and on my own outside therapy so I could report my success to my therapist. It felt too vulnerable to acknowledge my need for my therapist's help, and I feared being let down and disappointed as I had been in other relationships. It took a while for me to let down my façade of stoicism and self-sufficiency and reveal my scared, vulnerable self. But when I finally did, we began to make real progress.

From a therapist's perspective, we see the counseling relationship as foundational to everything else that happens in therapy. Counselors spend a lot of their training learning how to establish trust and begin well in the therapeutic process. Here are four essential practices you can expect your counselor to do in the initial phase of therapy to lay the foundations for a strong and trustworthy therapy relationship.

Practice 1: Counselors seek to understand your personal story and experiences. "Tell me why you are here" or "Tell me what brought you here today" is the question that begins most initial counseling sessions. As a psychologist, my primary intention for this first session is to invite the client to share their story of how they came to the place where they are seeking help. I will ask my clients about the problems that brought them into my office and the solutions they have tried, including the various ways they have sought help from family, friends, and other professionals. I am interested not only in the facts but also in how clients emotionally experience their problems. For example, the process of grief is a deeply individualized experience that I will want to understand both historically and emotionally from my client's perspective.

As clients tell their stories, therapists actively listen by clarifying questions, reflecting on what is heard, going deeper into some areas, and making connections. For therapists, our most important tool in the initial sessions is *empathy* as we seek to see the client's current problems through their own eyes, imagining what it would be like to be in their shoes. As we gain an empathic understanding of the problem, we reflect this back to the client to ensure we get it right. Our intent is to convey curiosity, respect, and positive regard for our client's experiences. Carl Rogers, the founder of person-centered therapy, describes the therapist's job in this way:

> When the other person is hurting, confused, troubled, anxious, alienated, terrified; or when he or she is doubtful of self-worth, uncertain as to identity—then understanding is called for. The gentle and sensitive companionship offered by an empathic person . . . provides illumination and healing. In such situations, deep understanding is, I believe, the most precious gift one can give to another.[7]

It is entirely normal to feel some anxiety about this first session. Clients often wonder: "Will I connect with the therapist? Will they understand me? Can I really talk about the struggles I've been having?" It can feel so awkward to unburden ourselves to a stranger. As therapists, we feel some anxiety, too, and we want to do everything in our power to create an atmosphere of safety, trust, and comfort for you so you can share your concerns openly, deeply, and honestly.

---

[7]Carl Rogers, *A Way of Being* (Boston: Houghton Mifflin, 1980), 160-61.

Practice 2: Therapists gather detailed information about the history of your current problems. In some ways, the initial session with a therapist shares commonalities with other medical visits in that it will involve an in-depth exploration of the current problem areas and how they developed. However, a therapist will also be interested in a more in-depth exploration of personal and family history to ensure that current issues are understood in the client's social, cultural, and religious context. For example, some clients may experience anxiety symptoms as an inevitable condition of living in a stressful world, while for others, these symptoms may feel like a shameful failure.

Therapists greatly appreciate when clients come to counseling sessions with any previous reflections and experiences that can help us understand their personal journey, such as journals, creative writing, artwork, or medical records from past treatments. We need you as clients to lead the way into a deeper understanding of your current concerns framed in the context of your past history. I always find it valuable to ask clients about any previous therapy experiences and what was helpful and not so helpful. This helps the client and me anticipate and navigate some of the normative challenges that occur in the helping relationship. For example, a client shared with me that he was not always sure what to talk about with his previous therapist and was confused about the goals of the work and how to make the best use of the therapy hour. I make sure to check in with him every couple of sessions about how our work is going and ask for feedback about his sense of progress and what to focus on in our sessions.

The goal of this first session is to develop a shared understanding of the current presenting problems that will form the basis of a collaborative treatment plan. I hope also to provide clients with a different view of their problems so they can begin to see potential solutions that they have not yet envisioned, that is, to activate hope.

Practice 3: Counselors provide a counseling agreement or informed consent. Whenever embarking on a new adventure, we are accustomed to reading about what to expect regarding risks, benefits, responsibilities, and guidelines. In counseling, we call this critical information *informed consent*.

Informed consent is foundational to establishing trust in therapy. At the outset, clients must be informed of the protections and rights that are the cornerstone of effective treatment. The initial session allows clients to ask questions and seek clarification before providing their agreement to enter into the therapeutic contract. Most therapists offer this information in a written document along with other forms where clients provide essential information. The forms and documents will include information about several key areas:

- *Risks and benefits of counseling.* Therapists describe how counseling can be beneficial for the client. While a successful outcome is not guaranteed, therapists agree to describe any risks involved with procedures, and clients are informed that they can end therapy at any time.

- *Confidentiality.* The content of therapy sessions, notes, assessment materials, and forms are all private health information protected by law. Therapists have an ethical responsibility to maintain client privacy. This means counselors cannot disclose anything about counseling sessions without written consent. There are limitations to this confidentiality if a client is a danger to themselves or someone else, or in the event of endangerment to a child or older adult, in which case a therapist is required to make a report to the appropriate authority.

- *Communication preferences.* Therapists will want to know what forms of communication are acceptable to clients (i.e., phone, text, email) and whether leaving a message or calling clients at work is okay. Some forms of communication are less private and secure than others, and clients need to know the risks to their privacy and consent to preferred communication mediums.

- *Telehealth.* If counseling includes telehealth sessions, the benefits and risks of telehealth will also be described, including therapist and client responsibilities. For example, most therapists will want the names of one or two emergency contacts in the event that a crisis occurs during a telehealth session and someone needs to be reached since the therapist is not physically present to help.

■ *Release of information.* If clients would like the therapist to coordinate their care with any other providers, such as a physician or psychiatrist, they will be asked to provide consent to release private health information. A consent form will specify what information the therapist can share with others and also specify how long the release of information is valid.

■ *Crisis.* The informed consent form will likely include information about the options in a crisis situation, including hotline numbers, how to reach the therapist, and usually instructions on going to the nearest emergency room in the event of a mental health crisis.

■ *Financial arrangements.* Informed consent includes the opportunity to clarify the cost, fees, and financial arrangements for counseling. If the therapist is filing insurance on the client's behalf, clients will need to permit their provider (or designee) to file insurance claims and release information, such as client diagnosis, as part of the claim process. With a fee-for-service financial arrangement, therapists provide a good-faith estimate of the total cost of psychotherapy, including an estimated length of treatment. It is important to clarify financial arrangements up front, so clients have realistic expectations about out-of-pocket expenses.

Practice 4: Therapists work with you to diagnose the problem and develop a treatment plan. As described in chapter one, mental health conditions often have multiple causes. For this reason, most counselors will take a detailed history of your current symptoms, including questions about medical history, physical and psychological symptoms, and potential triggers. Some therapists will ask clients to complete assessment measures such as a checklist of symptoms to gather important information about the presenting issues. Therapists will inquire in detail about the severity, duration, and frequency of symptoms to arrive at an accurate diagnosis of the presenting problem. The diagnosis will inform what interventions and treatment strategies are needed to alleviate the symptoms.

For many clients, it can be a great relief to know that symptoms and struggles have a name, are experienced by others, and have a pathway to treatment. However, there is always a risk that clients can experience a sense of stigma or shame when receiving a formal diagnosis or feel labeled in a way that is self-restricting or discouraging. To mitigate this risk of harm from diagnosis, I share with clients that diagnoses are primarily shorthand communication between professionals and that the label should in no way define or limit their views of self or hope for the future. While it can be sobering to be diagnosed with a mental health condition, it is an important first step toward accepting the need for help and engaging in the treatment process. Please know that as counselors, our work focuses on you as a person and not your diagnosis. If you have questions about how your therapist has arrived at a diagnosis, just ask.

YOUR MEDICAL RECORD

You may observe your therapist taking notes during your sessions and wonder what kind of records are kept regarding the counseling sessions. Like other health professionals, counselors maintain a medical record for each client that includes intake information, signed consent forms, assessment reports, treatment plans, and brief progress notes on each session. Most progress notes are relatively brief and limited to major issues discussed, treatment goals addressed, and treatment plans going forward. You have the legal right to review your medical record at any point during or following treatment.

Professional Ethics: Rules of the Road for the Counseling Journey

All licensed mental health professionals adhere to a code of ethics that provides regulations for the practice of psychotherapy and ensures protection for the public. The ethical codes are the professional guardrails for clients and therapists to enhance the safety and effectiveness of the counseling journey. Licensed mental health professionals affirm their commitment to professional ethics each time we renew our licenses. If clients believe their therapist has acted in an unethical or potentially harmful manner, they can file an ethics complaint with the state ethics committee or licensing board.

As therapists, our ethical commitments guide our actions and decision-making throughout the counseling process. We honor the public's trust in our profession and commit ourselves to providing services that benefit clients and cause no harm. We respect our clients' dignity, worth, and autonomy and preserve their confidentiality and privacy. We are committed to nondiscrimination and providing treatment for a diverse public with appreciation and acceptance of difference. As mental health professionals, we strive to uphold our responsibilities to clients and provide our services with excellence and integrity.

Because of the importance of the therapeutic relationship to the process and outcome of counseling, ethical guidelines exist for mental health professionals to help safeguard the relationship and ultimately protect the welfare of the client. These boundaries can seem rigid or inflexible at times, but they exist for the primary purpose of protecting the client and the effectiveness of the therapeutic process. Here are some common questions and scenarios that come up related to professional boundaries:

What kind of communication is possible between sessions? Ideally, between-session communication should be limited to phone calls, emails, or texts related to scheduling issues or should occur only in the event of a crisis or emergency. Talking with your counselor about what constitutes a crisis situation that necessitates between-session contact is beneficial. As counselors, we most often cannot provide the best help over the phone or via text/email, and it is ultimately better to discuss important issues during a regularly scheduled session. Scheduling an emergency session, if possible, is often a better solution than addressing issues over text or phone.

Is it possible to get together with my therapist outside our counseling sessions for social, ministry, or work-related reasons not related to my therapy? Ethically, counselors are committed to maintaining their professional role with clients and may not enter into a social relationship. In some settings, such as rural communities, it may be impossible for clients and therapists to avoid being involved in multiple roles with each other, as we may go to church together, know some of the same people socially, or run into each other at community events. While interactions outside counseling sessions may be unavoidable, the therapist must maintain confidentiality and take any necessary steps to ensure that the multiple roles are not harmful to the client or the therapeutic work.

What about social media? Similar guidelines apply to social media in terms of client-therapist engagement. While it is perfectly normal to be curious about your therapist, it is generally advisable not to seek a connection with your therapist via social media. Some professionals may have a separate social media platform for work- or ministry-related activities, and it is perfectly acceptable to engage with these venues.

Can I date my therapist? The short answer is no. It is highly unethical for therapists to engage in a dating, romantic, or sexual relationship with their clients. That being said, it is not unusual for clients to have feelings of attraction for their therapist, as it can be an emotionally intimate experience to be listened to and understood by another. Therapists can normalize these feelings for their clients while reaffirming and maintaining the professional boundaries of the relationship.

My therapist is great. Can I refer my friends and family members to them? It is the highest compliment when clients want to refer others to us. However, it is usually not a good idea to see multiple members from the same family for individual treatment (unless you are doing family therapy). Regarding seeing friends of current clients, the therapist and client should consider any potential impact on the therapeutic relationship before proceeding.

My therapy is drawing to an end. Can I transition to a social relationship with my therapist? It is difficult for therapists, too, to say goodbye at the end of a meaningful and productive therapy experience. However, it is important to preserve the professional relationship for a number of reasons. I will often tell clients that they have many friends but only one therapist and that my practice is to preserve the professional relationship in case they may want to return to therapy sometime in the future.

Faith Perspectives: The Therapeutic
Relationship as a Sacred Trust

As a Christian psychologist, I believe God has placed the innate need for secure and trusting relationships in the human heart. We are created in the image of a triune God who exists eternally as Father, Son, and Holy Spirit. Thus, in our very essence, we are created as relational beings. It is also good and right that our ultimate healing and wholeness are relationally mediated from our infancy through the end of our lives. It should come as no surprise that science has found evidence for what we know to be an eternal truth: relationships are foundational for healing.

Faith and trust are at the heart of the story of God's people. We see God initiating a trusting relationship with his people through the covenant he establishes with the people of Israel (Exodus 19:5-6) and then the ultimate, new covenant offered to all people through faith in Jesus Christ (Luke 22:19-20). The Israelites chose to put their trust in Yahweh and his appointed leader, Moses, to lead them through the wilderness into the Promised Land. As believers, when we put our trust in Christ, we enter into a relationship of secure and abiding love from which nothing can separate us (Romans 8:38-39) and begin the exciting adventure that is the Christian life. Our human fallibility in relationships, including the therapeutic relationship, is a far cry from this eternal and perfect love. Still, we are called to offer each other the kind of unconditional love and trust that God provides for each of us.

I am well aware of the difficult step it is for many clients to invest their time, money, and trust in therapy and risk hoping it will alleviate the pain and suffering they experience. As therapists, we view this investment in the therapeutic relationship as a sacred trust and do not take our professional or ethical responsibilities lightly. As a young therapist, I often felt the weight of this responsibility to clients and struggled with my own anxieties about whether I had enough knowledge and skills to truly help people. Over the years, I have grown to trust God's sovereignty and firmly believe that the clients he brings to me are divine appointments. I know many therapists feel the same. Even when the client and I decide we are not the right fit, I trust that we have learned something important from each other that will help in future relationships. As a Christian psychologist, I strive through the power of the Holy Spirit to offer clients my commitment to a trusting and secure, albeit imperfect, therapy relationship, including a desire to be aware of my shortcomings and repair relational disruptions.

I believe I can offer this sacred trust to clients because I know that God is active and present in the counseling office, guiding the psychotherapy process by the power of his Spirit and giving the gift of discernment to both the counselor and counselee. God's active presence is evident to me in many ways. I see God's provision of comfort when clients struggle to talk about seemingly intolerable, painful experiences. His gift of wisdom is evident during those aha moments when clients can make new connections and find freedom in life-changing insights. Over and over again, I have the privilege of bearing witness to God's gifts to clients as they faithfully endure suffering, courageously enact changes, and generously show mercy to others. I am confident that the client and I can trust in God's guidance and provision for all that is needed for the counseling journey.

Action Step: Building a Strong Relational Foundation

Clients also play a critical role in building a solid therapy relationship. As counselors, we need you as equal partners in building a foundation of trust for our future work together. Here are six actions steps that you can take to do your part to establish a collaborative, trusting relationship with your therapist:

1. Bring your questions, doubts, and concerns to the first session. Many clients have questions about the therapist's training and background, their specialty, and how long therapy will take, for example. As therapists, we welcome these questions and see them as evidence of your investment in the process.

2. Accurately report your symptoms and challenges, even when it feels embarrassing or shameful. Your honest response to questions

is critical in helping your therapist develop an accurate understanding of your problems and recommend an appropriate treatment plan.

3. Tell your therapist what has worked and not worked in the past. Knowing what went well and what went wrong with past therapy experiences is helpful so we can address these issues together.

4. Be honest about your needs and preferences for counseling. Remember, this is your treatment, specially customized for you! Treatment outcomes are significantly improved when clients are equal partners in developing a treatment plan that is individually suited to them.

5. Have patience with the process. Developing a solid therapeutic alliance takes time, and it is not uncommon for the first couple of sessions to feel a bit awkward as you and your therapist get to know each other and find a rhythm that works for you both. Remember also that most problems have taken a long time to develop, and if they were easily solved, you would have done so already.

6. Be curious and suspend judgment. I know, it's easier said than done. Voice your concerns and work with your therapist to customize the therapy to best suit your values and commitments.

As cliché as it may sound, it is absolutely true that the more you invest in building a strong therapy relationship, the more you will benefit from your counseling experience. Our fervent hope as therapists is that you are able to bring your honest and authentic selves to the therapy experience by voicing your anxieties, fears, preferences, and experiences. Trust that we, as therapists, are eager to partner with you to build the relational foundation that will prove essential for the counseling journey.

As I worked on this chapter to put into words the importance and process of building trust in therapy, I frequently found myself thinking of my experiences as a psychotherapy client. As someone who valued self-sufficiency, it probably took me longer than most to take emotional risks and trust my therapist. But now, when I think back on my therapy experiences, I remember very little about the theory or interventions my therapist used to encourage my growth. What I remember vividly, however, is my therapist's warm and attentive presence and their acceptance of the aspects of myself that seemed intolerable or shameful to let anyone see. This was the beginning of the healing journey for me.

Summing Up

Trust is an essential first step toward beginning well in therapy. As we start the counseling journey, we can remember that trust takes time as psychotherapy is a human encounter where both the client and therapist bring their hopes and fears. Ups and downs in the therapeutic relationship are inevitable as we repeat patterns in the therapy relationship that occur in our personal relationships. Still, relational ruptures can be repaired and only serve to strengthen the trust between client and therapist. Ultimately, we draw hope and courage from the certainty that God is active and present in the healing process.

Roles Recap: Beginning Well

THERAPIST ROLES	CLIENT ROLES
Establish a strong therapy relationship through active listening, empathy, respect, and genuineness	Tell your story with openness and authenticity; take risks and be open to developing a trusting relationship with your therapist
Explore the client's presenting problems and history, helping clients name and describe their current difficulties	Describe your issues and symptoms with honesty, accuracy, and specificity
Provide informed consent to clients regarding responsibilities and expectations for therapy	Articulate important worldview, cultural, and value commitments to incorporate into the therapeutic process
Abide by ethical commitments and boundaries to ensure the trustworthiness, safety, and effectiveness of treatment	Respect and honor therapeutic boundaries, asking questions when ethical concerns or issues arise

4

A User's Guide to Psychotherapy

Mapping Out the Counseling Process

*It seems like every therapist I see uses a different
approach, and I don't really know what they are aiming
for or what they expect from me in our sessions.*

A CLIENT'S REFLECTIONS
ON HIS THERAPY EXPERIENCE

*Client: Do we have to focus on my childhood in therapy?
I have so many problems in the here and now, and I'm
not sure how talking about the past will help.*

*Therapist: We can certainly focus on your concerns in the
here and now and bring in the past as needed to help us
understand the present issues. How does that sound?*

CLIENT AND THERAPIST EXCHANGE

For many, the experience of planning a trip is half the fun. We
spend hours diligently (and sometimes obsessively) poring over maps
and train schedules as we research potential destinations and how to
get there. Once we have completed our research, we can hopefully let
go and fully enter into the journey and even flex (okay, well, most of
the time) with the inevitable detours along the way. Similarly, I believe
that knowing what to expect from the counseling journey will empower clients to be active participants and gain the most from the
therapeutic experience. Even if you are more spontaneous and like to

take your travel journeys as they come, I encourage you to peruse this chapter to gain a lay of the land for the personal growth adventure we call therapy.

In this chapter, I will map out the therapeutic process, explore the various theories and approaches to psychotherapy, and offer nuggets of wisdom from the research regarding which approaches work best with specific problems. I will make a case for the assertion that there are many ways to reach the same destination and that the best route is one that we map out together as client and therapist, with the therapist serving as an expert guide to the process. Even when the journey encounters unexpected detours and roadblocks, clients and therapists work together from a foundation of trust to find the way forward. We start this chapter with a review of the various approaches to psychotherapy.

Counseling Theories 101: A Brief Overview of Approaches to Treatment

As an undergraduate student, I remember being drawn to the study of psychology as a fascinating science that explores how human beings develop, grow, and change. Psychological theories have contributed much to our understanding of mental health and how to bring about change through the counseling process. Each theoretical approach examines problems through a different lens and provides various counseling interventions for promoting growth and change. The various psychotherapy models can be thought of as different routes that lead to the same destination: improved mental health. Consider a map app on your smartphone, where you enter your starting point and destination and then see different routes to get you where you need to go, each way with different considerations such as side roads, tolls, and traffic slowdowns. Similarly, many therapeutic roads can lead you to your desired destination, and it is up to the client and therapist to determine the best route.

The therapist serves as an expert guide in the counseling journey and draws from their preferred theoretical models as well as research-based interventions to develop a treatment plan in collaboration with the client.[1] As a client, it is helpful to understand the road map the therapist is following to conceptualize and treat your presenting problems. If this is at all unclear, your job is to ask, "What approaches will we be using to address my problems, and how will they help?" The following section will look at the major models of psychotherapy and what you can expect from each approach. To illustrate the difference between approaches, we will consider how each model would approach the treatment of Lucia, a client who presents with symptoms of depression and low self-esteem.

Note: If the following discussion of counseling theories feels like too much detail for where you are right now, please feel free to skip ahead to "Common Factors" on page 75.

Psychodynamic psychotherapy. Doesn't any discussion of psychology inevitably lead back to Freud? While he is considered the father of the psychodynamic approach to therapy, this model of psychotherapy has come a long way since the days of the id, ego, and superego. Contemporary psychodynamic approaches share the view that current symptoms and difficulties result from our early relational experiences, which have a formative impact on how we view ourselves, significant others, and the world around us. Early injuries can result in unhealthy patterns of relating to others that are repeated into adulthood and create a repetitive cycle of unmet needs and psychological injuries. As these patterns are repeated in the therapeutic relationship, insights are gained, and a corrective emotional experience can occur. The primary mechanism of change with the psychodynamic approach is twofold: new *understanding* and new *experience*. Insight and awareness of these patterns and processes open the way for improved relational patterns to be developed and experienced, as corrective relational experiences enable clients to understand themselves in healthier, liberating ways.

Psychodynamic therapists will work with you to explore your relationship history and help you develop new insights about yourself and

---

[1] APA Presidential Task Force on Evidence-Based Practice, "Evidence-Based Practice in Psychology," *American Psychologist* 61, no. 4 (2006): 271-85, doi:10.1037/0003-066X.61.4.271.

your current difficulties, all in the context of a genuine and empathic therapeutic relationship. The relational growth and changes that happen in the therapy relationship will ripple outward into your other relationships, fostering health and flourishing.

Psychodynamic theories are a reminder of the importance of early emotional bonding experiences for human growth and development and provide insight into how individuals carry attachment-related needs and fears into adult relationships. We know from contemporary neuroscience findings on brain plasticity that, fortunately, attachment styles developed in childhood can be reworked and relearned in current relationships.[2] The psychodynamic approach is particularly effective for clients with long-standing personality and relational problems, and psychotherapy tends to be longer-term. There are also short-term contemporary psychodynamic approaches that have demonstrated effectiveness with a variety of issues, including depression and panic disorders.[3]

For our depressed client, Lucia, a psychodynamic approach would help her examine the contribution of her early experience to her current symptoms. Perhaps growing up in an alcoholic, neglectful home has contributed to a continued pattern of self-neglect and the belief that her needs and concerns do not matter to others, and this insight may help her begin to think and feel differently about herself. She may struggle to believe that her needs and concerns matter to her therapist, unconsciously repeating relational patterns from her early life. As she finds the courage to share this fear with her therapist, the therapeutic relationship provides the inroad to change her relational experiences with her therapist and others in her life, leading to stronger social connections and support.

Behavioral and cognitive-behavioral therapies. Psychological theories from the behavioral and cognitive-behavioral schools of thought

---

[2]Louis Cozolino, *The Neuropsychology of Psychotherapy: Healing the Social Brain*, 4th ed. (New York: W. W. Norton, 2017).

[3]Society of Clinical Psychology, "Research-Supported Psychological Treatments," American Psychological Association, https://div12.org/treatments/.

emphasize changes in thinking and behavior as the pathway to improved mental health. Behavioral approaches examine the ABCs of a situation: how Antecedents lead to Behaviors that lead to Consequences. Change the A or C, and you can change the behaviors. Behavioral approaches target changing the environment to change the outcome and are commonly used in parent training, milieu therapies (inpatient or residential programs with a reward-and-consequence system), and contemporary models such as dialectical behavior therapy, which helps clients develop behavioral stability and an improved ability to manage emotions.[4] Behavioral approaches are also effective with anxiety disorders and teach clients to utilize techniques such as progressive muscle relaxation, exposure to feared stimuli, and systematic desensitization.[5]

Similarly, cognitive-behavioral therapies target changing client's thoughts as the key to changing behavior and emotions. Clients learn to track their problematic thinking patterns, identify errors in thinking such as catastrophizing or overgeneralizing, and then correct their thinking with more accurate views of self and the world. In other words, cognitive-behavioral therapy retrains the brain to engage in more healthy and accurate thought patterns, interrupting negative patterns and fostering a more accurate and adaptive thought life.[6]

Contemporary cognitive-behavioral therapy approaches, often called third-wave cognitive-behavioral therapy, integrate mindfulness meditation with traditional cognitive-behavioral therapy practices to promote holistic well-being and growth. One popular example is acceptance and commitment therapy, which helps clients simultaneously accept their current symptoms (i.e., unwanted thoughts and feelings)

---

[4]For more information on dialectical behavior therapy, see Matthew McKay, Jeffrey C. Wood, and Jeffrey Brantley, *The Dialectical Behavior Therapy Skills Workbook: Practical DBT Exercises for Learning Mindfulness, Interpersonal Effectiveness, Emotion Regulation*, 2nd ed. (Oakland, CA: New Harbinger, 2019).

[5]Society of Clinical Psychology, "Research-Supported Psychological Treatments."

[6]Aldo Pucci, *The Client's Guide to Cognitive-Behavioral Therapy: How to Live a Healthy, Happy Life . . . No Matter What!* (n.p.: iUniverse, 2006).

while moving forward toward change strategies that align with their values and commitments.[7]

You can expect therapy sessions oriented toward cognitive-behavioral therapy to include education, in-session practice, and homework between sessions as new ways of thinking and behavior are introduced and encouraged to become part of your repertoire of habits and practices. With our depressed client, Lucia, cognitive-behavioral therapy would help her identify the negative thought patterns that may maintain her depressive symptoms and help her develop strategies to increase engagement in behavioral changes that will improve her mood, such as exercise, social interactions, and rewarding activities.

Behavioral and cognitive-behavioral therapy approaches have garnered much research support and are often considered the first-line treatments for anxiety, depression, phobias, and parent-focused treatment of childhood disorders, but they can also be applied to many other psychological conditions.[8]

Humanistic-experiential therapies. The third main school of psychotherapy encompasses humanistic-experiential approaches, which include person-centered, existential, emotionally focused, and positive-psychology approaches. Humanistic therapies share a high view of human potential for growth and development. These approaches also strongly emphasize developing an authentic and genuine therapeutic relationship as the primary vehicle for healing. Therapists often use in-session experiential techniques to help clients access their current emotional experiences.

Many therapists will describe themselves as *person-centered*, which is shorthand for an approach that highly values a genuine and collaborative relationship and seeks to personalize the counseling experience based on the client's needs and goals. Carl Rogers, the founder of person-centered therapy (also called client-centered therapy), believed that this relationship was both necessary and sufficient to promote

---

[7]For more information on acceptance and commitment therapy, see Steven C. Hayes, *Get Out of Your Mind and into Your Life* (Oakland, CA: New Harbinger, 2005).
[8]Society of Clinical Psychology, "Research-Supported Psychological Treatments."

client growth and wellness in therapy. Rogers advocated for a nondirective approach to therapy, where the therapist follows the client's lead, trusting that the client's natural inclination toward health will guide the process.[9] However, contemporary models suggest that a purely nondirective person-centered approach is not always efficient, and it is incumbent on the therapist to direct the therapy process to promote optimal growth. Within this model, the therapist is seen as the expert on the *process* of therapy to provide growth and change, while you as the client are the expert on your own *experience*, responsible for bringing to therapy your honest feelings, thoughts, and values.

Existentially oriented therapies hold similar values regarding the importance of the client-therapist genuine relationship but focus on exploring the *issues of existence* that are common to all human beings, such as meaning, existential isolation, death, and freedom.[10] Existential therapy is predicated on the theory that symptoms and difficulties arise when human beings encounter situations where they come face to face with the core issues of existence, evoking existential anxiety and defensive maneuvers to avoid the experience.[11] For example, I have worked with some clients who were able to pinpoint the onset of their symptoms to a milestone birthday, life transition, or significant anniversary that precipitated existential anxiety about their mortality and the meaning of their lives. By facing this anxiety directly in psychotherapy, they experienced relief from their symptoms and regained a sense of direction in their lives.

Emotionally focused approaches to therapy have gained popularity and impressive evidence for effectiveness with individuals, couples, and families. An emotionally focused therapist will help you slow your processing of experiences to allow deeper exploration of emotions and meanings. The therapist utilizes in-session enactments to help you bring your emotions into the here and now so they can be processed and understood. Emotionally focused therapies have demonstrated effectiveness for both individual and couple therapy. I have found that many

---

[9] Carl R. Rogers, *On Becoming a Person*, 2nd ed. (Boston: Houghton Mifflin, 1995).

[10] Irvin Yalom, *Existential Psychotherapy* (New York: Basic Books, 1980).

[11] Yalom, *Existential Psychotherapy*.

clients greatly value the opportunity to improve their emotional intelligence and awareness through this approach.[12]

A humanistic-experiential approach to Lucia's treatment would foster a deeper exploration of her experience of depressive symptoms, explore potential existential or grief-related precipitants, and use in-session interventions to help her express parts of herself that have been neglected or disowned toward strengthening the development of a more authentic self and improved relationships.

Family systems theory. A systems approach to understanding psychological symptoms views the problem as residing in the human system of relationships itself rather than the individuals involved. Families, organizations, and communities exhibit characteristic relational patterns, communication styles, and organizational structures that can contribute to developing or maintaining problems and symptoms. Treatment involves disrupting the system's homeostasis or balance and changing the dysfunctional patterns and structures, resulting in positive benefits for the individuals in that system. Think of a decorative mobile, where the hanging parts are interconnected through rods and string in a delicate balance. Pulling on one part of the mobile affects and mobilizes all the other components. The same is true of family systems: issues affecting one member affect the rest of the family. Accordingly, a treatment focused on strengthening the healthy characteristics of the system, such as boundaries, structure, and communications, can benefit the entire system.

The family systems approach to counseling and psychotherapy is often recommended as the best treatment choice for children, adolescents, and couples' issues. Systems approaches are also effective with a wide range of presenting problems such as eating disorders and chronic mental illness.[13] Even if you are pursuing individual psychotherapy, a

---

[12]For a more extensive discussion of this topic and a Christian appraisal of experiential therapies, see Terri S. Watson, Tracey Lee, Stanton Jones, and Richard Butman, "Experiential Psychotherapies," in *Modern Psychotherapies: A Christian Appraisal*, 2nd ed., ed. Stanton Jones and Richard Butman (Downers Grove, IL: InterVarsity Press, 2011), 291-345.
[13]Society of Clinical Psychology, "Research-Supported Psychological Treatments."

therapist may recommend that you invite significant others to the sessions to explore the presenting issues from a systemic perspective. We may discover in working with Lucia, for example, that conflictual interactions with her partner often precipitate her depressive episodes. A systems perspective would transition the treatment focus to relational patterns that may contribute to the maintenance of her depressive symptoms and may include her partner in therapy appointments.

Narrative or postmodern approaches to psychotherapy. These therapeutic approaches focus on how clients develop their personal narrative, including their understanding of themselves, their problems, and the world around them. Helping clients change the stories they tell themselves about their lives can shift their view of current problems, and new avenues for change and health can be envisioned. For example, Lucia's therapist may ask her to shift her focus away from her depressive symptoms to explore *exceptions* or situations in which these symptoms do not occur as a way of identifying her unrecognized strengths or resiliency. How might Lucia envision a life free of symptoms, and what would this look like? Changing the lens through which problems are viewed can open new ways of thinking and behaving that become improved strategies for living.

A therapist using a narrative approach will help you deconstruct the sociocultural factors that affect your views of self and others. You will develop a new script for your life that is not determined by your current problems or by internalized sociocultural stereotypes and biases. Postmodern therapies include narrative therapy, feminist therapy, and brief strategic family therapy. Many therapists find that integrating narrative therapy interventions with other approaches to therapy helps clients deepen their contextual understanding of their current issues.

Developmental models: Considering normative tasks and challenges. In addition to theories of psychotherapy, mental health professionals also rely on theories of psychosocial development as lenses to locate a client's current presenting problems in the context of their overall growth across the lifespan. For example, struggles with identity development would be expected in young adults but may be a contributing factor to Lucia's struggles if she is an older adult who is still very unsure about who she is and where her life is headed. Counseling can play a formative role in removing barriers to continued growth so that clients can continue to navigate the normative developmental tasks before them. Theories of human development abound, and the more sophisticated models focus less on stages of development, instead considering the interaction between individuals and their environment throughout the lifespan.[14]

As we wrap up this overview of the various theories your counselor may use, let me reiterate that the relationship you develop with your therapist has the most significant impact on the outcome of your therapy. Theory and interventions provide a valuable road map, but ultimately, *who* you travel with is more important than *how* you reach your destination. We will explore the science behind this truism in the next section.

Common Factors and Evidence-Based Psychotherapy: What Works for Whom?

Most therapists operate from an eclectic or integrative approach to psychotherapy rather than a single therapeutic orientation.[15] Practically, this means that a therapist will likely have a foundational theoretical orientation that guides their counseling work and then incorporate the most effective interventions across theoretical models that match a client's characteristics, preferences, and diagnosis. Mental health professionals are also trained to be research-informed in our clinical work, that is, to pay attention to the emerging science of psychotherapy and be knowledgeable about effective therapy's active ingredients. It is this integration of scientific knowledge in the context of an authentic human encounter that distinguishes the practice of psychotherapy from other health care interventions. As psychotherapy researchers Wampold and

---

[14]Urie Bronfenbrenner, *The Ecology of Human Development* (Cambridge, MA: Harvard University Press, 1979).

[15]Cristina Zarbo, Giorgio A. Tasca, Francesco Cattafi, and Angelo Compare, "Integrative Psychotherapy Works," *Frontiers in Psychology* 6 (2016): 2, doi:10.3389/fpsyg.2015.02021.

Imel articulate, "Something in the core of human connection and inter-action has the power to heal."[16]

Common factors research. The science of psychotherapy has come a long way in the past fifty years and has developed a robust evidence base. In the previous chapter, we reviewed the evidence that psychotherapy fosters significant improvement for clients experiencing various diag-noses and presenting problems. What is interesting about this research is that no one theoretical approach has been proven to be more effective across diagnoses. This has led to a body of evidence on the *common factors* across theories and therapies that lead to the best outcomes in treatment.[17] We know the primary importance of the therapeutic rela-tionship, as discussed in chapter three, as a common factor in effective psychotherapies. Other common factors that lead to good counseling outcomes include therapist empathy and respect for the client, therapist-client agreement on the goals and tasks of therapy, and the client's hope and positive expectancy that therapy will help them.[18] This important research reminds therapists that as enamored as we can get with psy-chological theories and techniques, we cannot lose sight of the fact that the psychotherapy relationship is what matters. As Irvin Yalom writes in *The Gift of Therapy*, "Therapy should not be theory-driven, but relationship-driven."[19]

Research-supported interventions. Another important question raised by psychotherapy effectiveness research is what works for whom, or which therapeutic approach will work best given the client's indi-vidual characteristics and diagnosis. In essence, therapists are en-couraged to develop a customized therapeutic approach for each patient, drawing from both theory and research.[20] Therapists engage in

[16]Bruce Wampold and Zac E. Imel, *The Great Psychotherapy Debate*, 2nd ed. (New York: Routledge, 2015), ix.
[17]Bruce Wampold, "How Important Are the Common Factors in Psychotherapy: An Up-date," *World Psychiatry* 14, no. 3 (October 2015): 270-77, doi:10.1002/wps.20238.
[18]Wampold, "How Important," 270-71.
[19]Irvin Yalom, *The Gift of Therapy* (New York: Harper Perennial, 2013), 20.
[20]John Norcross and Bruce Wampold, "A New Therapy for Each Patient: Evidence-Based Relationships and Responsiveness," *Journal of Clinical Psychology* 74, no. 11 (2018): 1891-93, doi:10.1002/jclp.22678.

continuing education throughout our careers to stay current on the research-supported interventions and strategies that are most effective in treating specific psychological conditions.[21] For example, research has demonstrated the value of incorporating some kind of exposure to feared stimuli as an essential element of treatments for various types of anxiety and trauma. How exposure therapy interventions are implemented will be based on specific client characteristics, preferences, and agreed-on therapy goals.

Why is this evidence base important? Knowing that a certain treatment has proven to be effective can strengthen the client's positive expectations that psychotherapy will help alleviate their distress and give them greater confidence in a good outcome. To illustrate, a client and I planned to use a specific protocol to treat his presenting problem. As he consulted with other medical professionals about his condition, they all suggested the same evidence-based treatment we planned to use. This high level of agreement between professionals strengthened the client's motivation and hope as we progressed with treatment, and ultimately, I believe, contributed to our good results.

Again, there are many routes to get to the same destination. It is essential that we keep in mind both research-supported interventions and the common therapy relationship factors throughout the entire therapy process to ensure the best outcomes. As a client, communicating with your therapist about your preferences, values, and goals will be an essential part of your therapy experience.

Faith Perspectives: Integration of Christian Faith with Psychological Theories

Psychological theories include value-based assumptions about how people grow, develop, change, and lead healthy and meaningful lives. Some theoretical assumptions may be based on philosophical perspectives that are inconsistent with a biblically based view of persons. For example, a behavioral psychology perspective will view human actions

---

[21]Society of Clinical Psychology, "Research-Supported Psychological Treatments."

as predetermined based on our biology and psychology interacting with environmental conditions. In comparison, Christian views of persons include foundational beliefs about the impact of free will, personal responsibility, sin, and grace on human behavior.

One of the tasks for Christian therapists and clients who want to integrate Christian faith and psychotherapy is to use a biblical and theological lens to evaluate the assumptions of psychological theories about personhood. This integrative work can take many forms. Christian scholars in psychology have thought long and deep about this endeavor, and there are many fine published works on a Christian evaluation of psychological theories.[22] Other scholars have adapted specific therapy approaches for application with Christian clients.[23] Counselors and clients can talk together about developing therapy goals and treatment plans that incorporate a Christian perspective on human growth, development, and life aims.

Another opportunity for faith integration involves incorporating spiritual practices and disciplines into all aspects of the therapy process, including assessment and intervention, and making meaning of suffering. In my practice, I explore clients' faith journeys and how their religious commitments may intersect with their current mental health concerns. Together, we identify spiritual practices that can enhance their use of psychological interventions. For example, I may teach a client struggling with anxiety to integrate deep breathing with a spiritual practice known as the breath prayer to help them seek God's presence moment by moment. Or I may recommend that a client practice a daily examen prayer to identify moments of blessing and gratitude. For clients from faith backgrounds that are different from my own, I will encourage them to incorporate meaningful spiritual practices into our work together. In this way, the therapeutic approach is adapted to the client's

---

[22]See, for example, Jones and Butman, *Modern Psychotherapies.*

[23]Examples include Joshua Knabb, *Faith-Based ACT for Christian Clients: An Integrative Treatment Approach*, 2nd ed. (New York: Routledge, 2022); and Sue Johnson and Kevin Sanderfer, *Created for Connection: The Hold Me Tight Guide for Christian Couples* (New York: Little, Brown, Spark, 2016).

religious and spiritual needs in a way that draws from the client's strengths and enhances treatment outcomes.

Developing a Treatment Plan: Your Personalized Road Map for the Counseling Journey

Treatment planning is a highly collaborative process between you and your therapist that involves identifying goals and desired outcomes with specific strategies for achieving each objective. Typically, your therapist will recommend an approach to treatment and the types of interventions that will work best to achieve your desired goals and provide an estimate of the frequency and duration of therapy. You are strongly encouraged to express your honest preference regarding treatment approaches, therapeutic activities, and your therapist's counseling approach.[24] As the treatment plan is executed, you will evaluate progress and provide feedback regarding your experience of therapy and progress toward your goals.

It is important for clients to agree with the treatment plan and understand how therapy can help them alleviate their current difficulties. This agreed-on understanding of the presenting problem and how therapy can help is valuable because it creates realistic expectations for counseling. With a road map for treatment, you can gain greater knowledge about what to expect and how to actively participate in the healing process.

Examples of treatment plans. Let's use our case example, Lucia, to illustrate a sample treatment plan for depression and low self-esteem. Through our assessment, we learned that Lucia's depressive symptoms, low self-esteem, and relationship challenges have been long-term issues for her. Lucia has identified the following goals for counseling: (1) to feel better about herself, (2) to experience less depression and more pleasure in life, and (3) to have better relationships with her spouse, children, and other family members.

---

[24]Joshua K. Swift, Jennifer L. Callahan, Mick Cooper, and Susannah R. Parkin, "The Impact of Accommodating Client Preference in Psychotherapy: A Meta-Analysis," *Journal of Clinical Psychology* 74, no. 11 (2018): 1924-37, doi:10.1002/jclp.22680.

In considering treatment approaches, the therapist recommends a short-term psychodynamic approach to psychotherapy as an approach that has good research support in treating Lucia's symptoms and is consistent with her goals. Lucia and her therapist develop a treatment plan that includes weekly individual therapy to (1) foster insight into how Lucia's past experiences affect her view of herself, (2) improve her ability to identify and express emotions, and (3) explore her relational patterns and triggers that lead to withdrawal and disengagement with others. The therapist predicts six to eight months as the estimated length of treatment.

For another example, we can consider what a possible treatment plan would look like for our client from chapter two, who experiences acute anxiety symptoms that interfere with their ability to work. Goals for this client may include (1) learning practical skills for dealing with anxiety symptoms and panic attacks, (2) understanding why panic attacks happen, and (3) getting back to work with fewer sick days due to anxiety symptoms.

A therapist with this client will likely use an approach to therapy that includes both cognitive and behavioral elements. Cognitive-behavioral therapy for panic disorders is an evidence-based approach that a therapist may recommend for this client. The client and therapist develop a treatment plan together for weekly psychotherapy focusing on (1) identifying and managing anxiety triggers; (2) learning coping skills, including relaxation and mindfulness skills; (3) eliminating avoidance behaviors through graduated exposure to feared stimuli; and (4) joining an online group for clients struggling with anxiety for psychoeducation and support. The estimated length of treatment is likely to be three to six months.

Some therapists prefer a less structured approach to treatment planning, relying on a preferred theoretical approach and the interventions that they have found to be generally effective with the issues that clients typically bring to therapy. For example, a counselor with a person-centered or psychodynamic approach may focus on the client's experience of their problems in the here and now and less on teaching skills to promote behavioral change. If this is the case, it is still valuable for clients to gain a general understanding of the therapist's mental road map for psychotherapy and to have the opportunity to provide feedback and input on the direction of therapy. As therapists, we need to do a better job of informing clients about our beliefs and assumptions about the psychotherapy process, including naming and describing the theoretical approach and techniques we believe will be helpful to them. This is an essential aspect of informed consent and also builds trust with clients as we invite their active participation in charting a course for their therapy experience.

Adapting therapy to your cultural, community, and worldview commitments. Psychotherapy research has taught us that adapting treatment approaches to align with the client's characteristics and culture leads to the best therapeutic outcomes.[25] Cultural adaptation of treatment includes exploring with the client the aspects of their cultural worldview and values that inform their view of health and well-being. For example, a client who values altruism as an indicator of health and maturity will benefit from treatment approaches and goals that link therapy interventions to serving others as an essential outcome.

Customizing treatment to the client's personal context is enhanced when clients can share their important cultural values openly and honestly with the therapist and feel that the therapist seeks to understand and respect them. It is the therapist's job to inquire about your cultural values and explore the potential implications of demographic differences between you. However, it is equally important that you speak up if you feel that a therapeutic approach or intervention may be in tension with your values.

To illustrate, let's say our client above, Lucia, would like to incorporate faith-based practices and spiritual disciplines into her counseling work. Customizing her treatment plan may include adding guided prayer exercises, meditating on Scripture to help her develop a more biblically based view of herself, and joining a Bible study at her church for support and fellowship.

---

[25]Norcross and Wampold, "New Therapy," 1891-93.

Summing Up

As we come to the end of this chapter, I hope the process of therapy and how clients can actively participate has been demystified. Many therapeutic routes can lead to improved well-being and symptom relief as clients and therapists work together to customize a treatment plan that best fits the client's presenting problems and personal context. Effective therapists, in other words, create a new and unique therapy for every client.[26] Proactive and engaged clients (this is you!) seek to be well-informed about where their counseling journey is headed and share their input, feedback, and preferences all along the way.

It may feel daunting to pull back the curtain of the therapy experience and consider the various theories and research that guide the counseling process. Remember that research has found that the trusting relationship you form with your therapist is more important than which theory they use. Therapists who are collaborative, responsive, and flexible, and who seek feedback from clients will provide effective counseling regardless of their preferred theory.[27] A sensitive and skilled counselor will work with you to develop a personalized treatment plan, respond to your questions, and continually seek feedback about how the process is going for you.

At the beginning of the book, I likened the counseling process to the exodus of the people of Israel through the wilderness. Indeed, the wilderness is humbling (and sometimes terrifying) for those of us who anticipate that a well-structured map and plan can always lead directly to our desired destination. As useful as psychological theory, interventions, and treatment planning are to the counseling process, I encourage you to prepare for the unexpected in your counseling experience. Like any journey, it is often the surprises and detours along the way that, in the end, will be the most transformative part of the process.

---

[26]Norcross and Wampold, "New Therapy," 1891.

[27]John C. Norcross and Michael J. Lambert, "Psychotherapy Relationships That Work III," *Psychotherapy* 55 (2018): 303-15, https://doi.org/10.1037/pst0000193.

Roles Recap: Mapping Out the Counseling Process

THERAPIST ROLES	CLIENT ROLES
Apply knowledge from theory and research to understand the client's presenting problems	Share openly in sessions about pressing issues and concerns
Collaborate with the client to identify goals and develop a treatment plan	Collaborate with a therapist to identify goals and develop a treatment plan
Adapt the therapeutic approach to the client's individual culture and context	Articulate important worldview, cultural, and value commitments
Incorporate a biblical worldview and spiritual practices into the approach to therapy for interested clients	Inform your therapist if you are interested in including spiritual practices as part of your treatment plan

5

You Are Here

How to Gain the Most from Your Psychotherapy Experience

Therapist: We have been meeting together for about eight weeks, and I wanted to take some time during our session to review our treatment plan and discuss the progress you feel you have made toward your goals. I'd also really value your feedback on the counseling process—what has been helpful and not so helpful, and are there any changes we need to make going forward?

Client: It's been great, you've been really helpful, and I definitely feel that I'm making progress. . . .

Therapist: Sounds like there's a "but" in there. . . .

Client: I had hoped that my depression would be lifted by now and it is just sobering to face that it is harder to change than I thought. I am feeling kind of stuck and not sure what to talk about in our counseling sessions.

Therapist: Let's spend some time talking about this in our session today.

The last chapter provided an overview of the therapy process, describing how counselors draw from psychological theory and research to work with clients to develop a customized road map for the counseling journey. This chapter is about making the journey your own. As a client, you have the power and the responsibility to ensure that the psychotherapy process is just what you need it to be for your growth and development. Yes, you will benefit significantly from the guidance of a skilled and trusted therapist-guide. But if we think about it, the specifics of the journey are really up to you, including what you talk about in therapy, the work you do between sessions, and how honest you are with your therapist. Your counseling journey does not belong to your spouse, mother, father, friends, or even your therapist; it is your own. *You are here*—on your own counseling journey. How are you going to make the most of it?

This chapter is chock-full of practical strategies and recommendations for gaining the most from your therapy experience. It includes what your therapist wants you to know about your essential part in the process to empower you to play an active role in treatment. We will delve into insights for making the most of your therapy hour, right-sizing your expectations for therapy, and accelerating momentum through between-session work. Finally, we will look at a checklist for creating the optimal environmental conditions to support your growth journey. Let's dive right in.

The Therapy Hour

The counseling journey takes place one session at a time, so the first order of business is to determine how best to use that precious hour that makes up each leg of the counseling journey. Your treatment plan and goals provide general guidance for the focus of therapy. But, as a client, it is largely up to you to decide what you talk about, how honest you are with your therapist, and your here-and-now engagement during the hour. The following suggestions provide guidance on making the best use of your counseling sessions.

What should I talk about in therapy? Most clients find it helpful to think ahead of time about how they want to use their session and what topics they would like to address. I will often suggest to clients that their job is to bring the *content* to the sessions, including the important thoughts, feelings, and behaviors related to their presenting problem, while my job is to guide the *process* of therapy toward achieving our agreed-on goals.

Typically, I encourage clients to talk in session about the issues that weigh heaviest on them, such as the places where they feel stuck, uncomfortable, distressed, or even ashamed. The emotional intensity around a topic is often a trustworthy guide that an issue could benefit from being processed in therapy. Any patterns you notice in your day-to-day life and relationships are also grist for the therapy mill. It is worth paying attention when a significant other, a friend, or a colleague says, "Maybe you should talk about this with your therapist."

The specific content of counseling sessions will vary depending on the type of therapy used. Some therapeutic approaches are highly structured with a particular protocol for the therapy hour. For example, a cognitive-behavioral approach such as acceptance and commitment therapy or dialectical behavior therapy will likely include a discussion of homework assigned the previous week, teaching and practicing new skills in session, and a homework assignment for the next week. A family systems therapist may ask a couple or family to talk with each other about a recent problematic interaction and then provide relational coaching to help the family identify and restructure relational patterns.

With other approaches, such as psychodynamic and humanistic-experiential therapies, the therapist may begin the session by checking in with the client on any thoughts or feelings that came up during the week in response to the last session. Then the client talks about the issues and concerns most on their mind. The therapist listens empathically and looks for opportunities to foster insight, make connections, and encourage deeper exploration consistent with the agreed-on goals for therapy. A significant part of the education and training of therapists involves helping counselors know how to listen and where to intervene to promote psychological health. As hard as it can be, you can trust the process by speaking honestly and openly about your concerns, knowing that your therapist is listening empathically and skillfully.

Some clients may find it challenging to convey their thoughts and feelings with words. Many counselors incorporate expressive therapy techniques such as art, creative writing, role-plays, and psychodrama into the therapeutic process to help clients with self-expression. Part of customizing the therapy experience for each client is finding the most helpful mode of expression for feelings and fears that are hard to put into words. If you find it difficult to use your words, do not be discouraged. Ask your therapist about possible expressive therapy techniques that can help you convey what is on your mind and heart.

The benefits of honest and vulnerable disclosure. One of the curative factors of the therapeutic process occurs as clients share themselves fully with another person and receive empathy, acceptance, and support. Through this process, clients can move toward greater understanding and acceptance of the disowned parts of themselves to great benefit. In *Secrets and Lies in Psychotherapy*, the authors describe the benefits of honest disclosure in this way:

> The central task of therapy is to facilitate clients' ability to disclose and ultimately accept previously hidden and shameful parts of themselves. The syllogism is deceptively simple: Clients hide what they cannot accept; with the therapist's help, they disclose that which they have previously found unacceptable; their disclosure leads to acceptance; and their acceptance leads to change.[1]

Bringing hidden feelings, fears, experiences, and thoughts into the light takes great courage but brings many benefits. One meaningful example of this was a client who shared her most carefully guarded secret with me, only to marvel at the relief she experienced afterward. When I asked her what it was like to share this with me, she revealed that she had imagined that I would recoil from her with rejection or possibly run from the office in horror. Bringing this hidden part of herself into the light alleviated her shame and fostered a more curious and accepting attitude toward these aspects of her life and experience.

Much within us resists honest disclosure, and some aspects of our experience have remained hidden for a reason. It is not uncommon for clients to want their therapist's approval and acceptance so much that they share only selective aspects of their story in therapy, particularly in the beginning of the treatment process when the therapy relationship is still

---

[1]Barry Farber, Matt Blanchard, and Melanie Love, *Secrets and Lies in Psychotherapy* (Washington, DC: American Psychological Association, 2019), 58.

being formed. While most clients are generally honest with their therapist (as it is undoubtedly self-defeating not to be!), research on secret-keeping in psychotherapy has found that nearly two-thirds of all clients do not reveal important information to their therapist that could make a difference in their therapy. Client secret-keeping most often occurs in the following areas: severity of symptoms, sexual content, substance abuse, trauma history, and feelings about the therapist or progress in therapy.[2]

In any human relationship, there are many reasons why it is difficult for people to reveal all aspects of themselves to another. It should come as no surprise then that even in a confidential, professional counseling relationship, clients conceal or do not share information for fear that their therapist will not understand, overreact, or be hurt or angry. Some issues can just feel too overwhelming to discuss. However, it is notable that the harder an issue is to bring up in therapy, the more critical it is that you find the courage to speak about it, as it will have a high likelihood of contributing to the healing process.

Therefore, we can add one more rule of thumb for getting the most out of the therapy process: make every effort to talk with your therapist about the issues that are most difficult to discuss. Just as the intensity of feelings can be a marker of the importance of an issue to the therapy process, the intensity of desire to avoid can indicate a significant topic for the therapy hour.

Here-and-now focus. One substantive way counseling sessions differ from social interaction is the focus on here-and-now experiences. Clients can often faithfully recount their experiences outside the therapy office with fear-inducing situations, challenging relationships, and emotional triggers. However, bringing those experiences into the here and now of the therapy office provides significant opportunities for progress toward goals. For example, treatment for anxiety and phobia reactions may involve asking clients to imagine themselves in the anxiety-producing situation and then directing the client to employ relaxation

---

[2]Matt Blanchard and Barry Farber, "Lying in Psychotherapy: Why and What Clients Don't Tell Their Therapist About Therapy and Their Relationship," *Counselling Psychology Quarterly* 29, no. 1 (2016): 90-112, https://doi.org/10.1080/09515070.2015.1085365.

strategies in the session to manage the anxiety. Experiential therapy techniques, such as the empty-chair technique, can help clients deal with unfinished business with significant others even without the person present, through envisioning and enacting important conversations in the therapy office. In couples therapy, therapists help clients express to each other in the session the relational needs and fears that drive their interpersonal dance so that new patterns of interaction can occur.

The problematic relational dynamics in a client's life will also be enacted in the therapy office as we repeat our relational patterns in the here and now. For example, a client who has difficulty forming trusting relationships with others will likely employ similar strategies to keep the therapist at a distance, often without awareness that the very problems the client is seeking treatment for are being enacted with the therapist. Rather than an impasse, these repetitions are excellent opportunities for here-and-now work as the therapist respectfully and sensitively brings the enactment to the client's attention. For example, I brought to a client's attention that he would regularly change the subject whenever our sessions began to focus on his areas of vulnerability, a dynamic that I suspected happened frequently in his closest relationships to keep people at a safe distance. While it was a little anxiety-provoking at first, the here-and-now focus soon became a valuable part of our therapy work and provided real-time opportunities for us to understand and address these relational patterns in his life.

For therapy to be truly effective, clients also need to be able to take the gains they have made in the therapy office and apply the new knowledge and skills they have learned to their lives outside therapy. Thus, there is a rhythm to the therapeutic process: your life experiences are brought into the here and now in the therapy office, where insight and change can occur, and then these changes can be applied to your daily life.

Modifying Expectations: What Will Probably Not Happen in Therapy Sessions

While every counseling journey is unique, certain types of interactions will likely not occur in counseling and may even be counterproductive.

Sometimes this can be surprising or disappointing to clients who expect something different. In this section we look at some types of interactions that will likely not occur in therapy and why they can be detrimental.

A quick fix. Sometimes, clients begin psychotherapy with the expectation that the experience will mirror a visit to a physician's office with a single-session diagnosis and treatment of the presenting problem. However, the complexity of mental health issues requires a different kind of approach, where the therapist and client are co-collaborators in assessment, diagnosis, and treatment direction. I like to tell clients that if the causes and solutions to their psychological issues were easy to determine, they would have already figured it out for themselves without the help of therapy!

This is not to say that psychotherapy is always a long-term endeavor. The duration of the counseling process and frequency of sessions depends on several factors, including the type and severity of symptoms, how long the client's problems have been going on, and the goals for therapy. Early studies on length of treatment found that half of all clients report a decrease in symptoms by eight sessions, while three-fourths of clients indicate significant improvements at the twenty-six-session mark.[3] Some clients choose to continue in therapy once their initial distress has been alleviated to work on additional issues. Others may finish their course of treatment with the plan to return at a future date if problems resurface. Evaluation of treatment duration and effectiveness is an ongoing part of the therapeutic process, and you and your therapist will likely determine the length of treatment and frequency of sessions collaboratively.

Advice giving. Clients come to therapy because they have tried many solutions to complicated problems. The idea behind the treatment is not to see an expert who will fix your problem by giving directive advice but to work collaboratively with someone who can help you find

---

[3]Kenneth I. Howard, S. Mark Kopta, Merton S. Krause, and David E. Orlinsky, "The Dose-Effect Relationship in Psychotherapy," *American Psychologist* 41, no. 2 (1986): 159-64, https://i-cbt.org.ua/wp-content/uploads/2017/11/Howard-dose_effect-psychotherapy-1986.pdf.

personalized solutions to your presenting concerns. A therapist's education and training involve a variety of approaches to promoting change that may include teaching coping skills, exploring secondary gains to problem behaviors, and generating potential solutions. However, a good therapist will rarely tell clients what to do.

This is because you are the expert on your own life and circumstances (while it certainly does not feel that way to clients sometimes!). Your personal perspective is of paramount importance, and it is difficult for counselors to truly grasp all of the complexities involved in your life decisions. As counselors, we can help you explore, weigh, and choose the best solution to your problems, empower you to act, and then help you evaluate the outcome to inform your decisions in the future. You will then have the satisfaction of knowing that you are the one who can bring about changes in your life, with the support of your therapist. In the end, this will increase your sense of personal agency and self-confidence. I find that a successful outcome to therapy includes my client's realization that they have been the primary author of their own healing and recovery success story.

Focusing primarily on other people. Sometimes clients will devote their time in therapy to talking about the significant others in their lives and how they contribute to their current difficulties. Assessing the impact of relationships on the client's presenting concerns is an integral part of the treatment process. However, it is counterproductive if counseling sessions focus primarily on others and how they need to change. The best use of psychotherapy is to focus on how clients are affected by challenging people in their lives, as well as their own contributions to their problems and how they can respond to significant others in new and improved ways. Often, clients will use therapy to vent their frustrations with the people in their lives, which is expected. However, a good therapist will help you move beyond focusing on changing others to a place of personal responsibility and recognition of what you can do to change yourself.

An important exception to a focus on personal responsibility is when the client is experiencing harm at the hands of others in abusive, neglectful, or discriminatory relationships and environments. In situations where there is domestic violence, bullying, or workplace harassment or discrimination, for example, the therapist will likely focus on advocacy and empowerment strategies that help the client protect themselves from the harmful behavior of others. In situations involving harm, it is counterproductive and even detrimental for clients to engage in self-blame and take on the responsibility for the abusive behavior of another person.

Therapists talking about themselves. Counseling is one place where clients receive the benefit of focusing on their own thoughts, feelings, and experiences without the need for reciprocal interest in another, as is common in social interactions. While clients are often curious about their counselor's personal life and experience, too much therapist self-disclosure shifts the focus away from the client and is inappropriate for the counseling process. Therapist self-disclosure should always be used judiciously and in the service of helping the client. Revealing aspects of our lives to clients can help to humanize the therapeutic encounter and underscore that we, too, are not immune from problems and challenges. However, maintaining a focus on you as the client is paramount for effective psychotherapy.

Focusing on the facts alone (versus how they make you think and feel). Another aspect of therapy that is quite different from social interaction occurs when clients share stories and experiences related to the presenting problem. In social interactions, this sharing often involves telling stories from beginning to end with specific descriptions and details related to a given experience. In psychotherapy, the focus is on slowing down the narrative to explore more deeply how an experience evokes specific thoughts, feelings, and behaviors. A cognitive-behavioral therapist will want to unpack a situation to help you understand the trigger event, the resulting thought, and the emotional and behavioral response. A relational or psychodynamic therapist will want to explore how your experience may seem familiar to past situations. Experiential therapists will help you deepen your emotional experience of an interaction to understand its meaning and significance.

All of these levels of inquiry require the therapist to interrupt your story, slow it down, and refocus your attention on important aspects of your experience that require further exploration, much like shifting a video replay into slow motion. At times, this can feel disconcerting to clients if they cannot recount the facts of their entire story. Be assured that your therapist is listening carefully for intervention points to help you make sense of your experience in a way that will open up new insight, emotional awareness, and possibilities for responding differently to life events. As therapists, we want to make the best use of the therapy hour to help clients achieve their stated goals, and this may require a new and different way for clients to reprocess their stories.

Faith Perspectives: Practicing Presence During the Therapy Hour

One of the greatest gifts of the therapy session is that it offers a transitional, in-between space where you can leave the familiar behind and consider the hoped-for future that has not yet been obtained. In the counseling room, you step out of your day-to-day experience to reflect on your life, considering where you have been and where you want to go. With your phone silenced and laptop closed, you are invited to press pause on the activities of daily living to deeply explore who you are and who you hope to become. Like the wilderness journey metaphor we considered at the beginning of the book, the therapy experience invites you to let go of the familiar and be open to new and unexpected opportunities for growth and transformation.

Recently, in a conversation with a friend, we discovered how much we both enjoyed the experience of traveling by airplane. We agreed that something about being suspended in the air between destinations, unreachable by phone, text, or email, puts both of us in a reflective mood. I think it is the fact that plane journeys are a kind of transitional, liminal space where daily demands are suspended for a time that creates room for quiet contemplation. The therapy hour can also be a liminal space where we can quiet ourselves to be especially attuned to God's presence, love, and guidance.

I believe the sacred space created in the counseling room allows clients to find the courage to speak the truth of all that is in their hearts and minds, even the old hurts and embarrassing secrets that haunt them. With the support of a trusted counselor and guide, clients journey into the pain and suffering of unprocessed experiences in search of deeper understanding and new meanings. They can grow, learn, grieve, lament, hope, aspire, accept, and change in this liminal space. Psychotherapy can be a sacred and transformative experience where we carve out the space and time in our lives to talk about what really matters.

What are the necessary ingredients for psychotherapy to become such a transitional experience? I offer two recommendations: *preparation* and *presence*. Just as you prepare for an airplane journey with a backpack of water, snacks, and reading material, it is beneficial to prepare for the counseling session and bring what is needed to allow yourself to be fully present. It can be helpful to review the week before your therapy session and consider what thoughts, feelings, or experiences arose that were significant and beneficial to process further. Sometimes, clients prefer to arrive early to spend a few minutes in the waiting room to consider what they need to discuss and to prepare themselves mentally, emotionally, and spiritually for the therapy session. Many of my clients enjoy the ritual of making cups of hot tea and getting out their journals before settling into the chair or couch in my office to begin our session. If you are working with your therapist via telehealth, it is especially important to carve out preparation time for yourself before you click on the link to begin your session.

The second essential ingredient for transformative psychotherapy is to develop the capacity to be *fully present* during the therapy hour. This practice comes easily for some but may be more difficult for others. Ideally, you will want to schedule your therapy appointment when you can step away from responsibilities and distractions. If possible, you will want to silence your phone and turn off notifications during your sessions. Some clients find it beneficial to begin the session with a breathing or visualization exercise or a prayer to shift their focus to the therapy hour.

How do we attune ourselves to God's presence during the therapy hour? In the devotional classic *Practicing the Presence of God*, seventeenth-century monk Brother Lawrence describes the practice in this way: "I make it my priority to persevere in His holy presence, wherein I maintain a simple attention and a fond regard for God, which I may call an actual presence of God. Or, to put it another way, it is a habitual, silent, and private conversation of the soul with God."[4]

This contemplative practice can be challenging if you are experiencing distress and feeling distant from God. However, Brother Lawrence offers words of encouragement to persevere when God seems far away:

> You need not cry very loud. He is nearer to us than we are aware. And we do not always have to be in church to be with God. We may make an oratory of our heart so we can, from time to time, retire to converse with Him in meekness, humility, and love. Every one is capable of such familiar conversation with God, some more, some less. He knows what we can do.[5]

Practicing the presence of God during therapy hour can become a precious and life-giving spiritual experience for both clients and therapists, one that we will aspire to continue moment by moment in our daily lives.[6]

Action Steps: Building Momentum Through Between-Session Work

Change is hard work and requires the investment of time and effort beyond the psychotherapy hour. Following through on between-session homework is essential for the transformative change of long-standing habits of thinking, feeling, and behaving. As is the case with many journeys, the character-forming practices and habits we learn along the

---

[4]Brother Lawrence, *The Practice of the Presence of God* (2002), available at www.gutenberg .org/cache/epub/5657/pg5657.txt.
[5]Brother Lawrence, *Practice of the Presence*.
[6]For an excellent discussion of contemplative practices to integrate with therapy, see Joshua Knabb, *Faith-Based ACT for Christian Clients: An Integrative Treatment Approach*, 2nd ed. (New York: Routledge, 2022).

way can be even more important than the arrival at our destination and will help us deal with problems and challenges in the future.

Counseling homework can take many forms depending on the therapeutic approach and goals. Behavioral and cognitive-behavioral homework includes activities such as keeping thought records, practicing skills, or trying out new ways of thinking and behaving. Therapists using an experiential or emotion-focused approach may give you *attention homework*, requesting that you pay attention to various feelings and experiences that come up throughout the week, including the triggers and resulting feelings. A systems approach may encourage you to pay attention to *relational patterns* and take steps to change conflictual cycles, for example. Whatever the assignment, between-session work is essential for transferring the gains you are making in therapy to your day-to-day life.

One caution to remember about between-session work is that the very symptoms clients enter therapy to deal with can create challenges for following through with homework assignments. A depressed client may struggle with a sense of hopelessness and helplessness, believing nothing they do will make a difference. An anxious client may worry about doing the homework wrong or disappointing their therapist. When the inevitable barrier occurs to completing between-session work, it becomes an opportunity to delve deeper into the obstacles that get in the way of growth and change. Even when you cannot successfully complete between-session homework, processing the experience with your therapist can yield essential information about why your problems seem so sticky and immovable.

Here are some high-impact activities you can do between sessions to build momentum toward change and growth. Please do not feel like you must do them all! Make note of the recommendations that are most inviting and relevant for you right now.

Journaling. An invaluable between-session activity involves carving out time during the week for self-reflection and journaling. When we journal, we draw from the insights of our own inner therapist to make sense of our lives and in doing so strengthen our self-reflective muscles.

There are many options for journaling in addition to the traditional writing practice. I have clients who record voice memos for themselves or even create private accounts on social media platforms to keep a record of their thoughts and experiences. Other clients write poetry, create art, or compose music as a form of self-expression for the insights gained throughout the counseling journey. An added benefit of journaling is that your writings and recordings will become an invaluable archive of your counseling journey that you can look back on in the future.

Bibliotherapy. Reflective reading can also enhance the counseling experience. Bibliotherapy is a form of therapy often used as a complementary treatment alongside traditional psychotherapy, where clients use reflective reading of poetry, novels, and self-help books for personal growth. Clients can search for reading resources independently and also ask their therapist for recommendations. Insights gained from bibliotherapy can be integrated into the therapeutic process, just like you are doing right now as you read this book!

Trying out new insights and actions in relationships. One of the best resources for clients is their social support network, where they can share insights and gains made in therapy with their family, friends, and even coworkers. Talking with others about the changes happening within yourself helps you solidify growth areas and enact new ways of thinking, feeling, and behaving in your daily life and relationships. Plus, it is the best advertisement for getting your friends and family to pursue their own therapy as they see the benefits you have gained.

HOW MUCH SHOULD I SHARE WITH FRIENDS, FAMILY, AND COLLEAGUES?

Your counseling journey is your own, and it is entirely your choice if you choose to share any information with others about your psychotherapy. However, it can bring significant benefits to the therapy process to take the gains you are making in the therapy office and incorporate them into your day-to-day life and relationships. As you begin to make connections, develop insight, and try out new behaviors, you may inevitably want to share your experiences with others and potentially gain their support for the process. You will want to balance your right to privacy with your need for support from others during your mental health journey.

The question may be less about *whether* you share and more about *who* you share your journey with. My encouragement is to share openly with close family and friends who will be able to provide a supportive presence during the journey. With others, including work colleagues and acquaintances, you may want to decide on a case-by-case basis whether and how much you want to share.

Sharing about your therapy experience with others may also provide opportunities for feedback and for asking for support, and sometimes can normalize your experiences, as friends often respond with, "I've felt that way too!" Hopefully, as those around you get to know you in deeper and more human ways, your connections will strengthen as a source of mutual support.

Mental health apps for phones or computers. In recent years, there has been a proliferation of mental health apps for phones and computers that provide extra support for therapeutic goals and interventions. Apps can support the change process by providing education, behavioral tracking, skills training, and even therapeutic games. Many approaches to therapy have corresponding phone and computer apps that can help clients throughout the therapy process. I frequently recommend various apps to clients to support their between-session work and help them bring the skills they learn in therapy into their daily lives. Clients appreciate the easy access to these resources on their phones, and many basic apps can be used free of charge.

Altruism and volunteer work. During the counseling journey of introspection and self-discovery, caring for others can provide an important balance. Research has demonstrated the mental health benefits of altruistic actions, which boost positive mood and provide a sense of meaning.[7] We can improve our care for others even as we learn to better care for ourselves. I will sometimes encourage clients to find an activity

---

[7]Sarah D. Pressman, Tara L. Kraft, and Marie P. Cross, "It's Good to Do Good and Receive Good: The Impact of a 'Pay It Forward' Style Kindness Intervention on Giver and Receiver Well-Being," *Journal of Positive Psychology* 10, no. 4 (2015): 293-302, doi:10.1080/17439760.2014.965269.

or cause that has personal significance, such as community service or church volunteer work. As clients move through the healing process, volunteer support for others struggling with similar issues can be especially meaningful. Twelve-step programs are an excellent outlet for giving back what we have learned, as those further along in their recovery become sponsors and supporters of others who are earlier in the process.

Spiritual disciplines. For clients who are interested in integrating their faith into their counseling experience, engaging in spiritual practices and habits between sessions encourages holistic spiritual and psychological growth. Scripture study, prayer, worship, confession, and practicing Sabbath are spiritual disciplines that God uses as part of our sanctification process of growth into spiritual maturity. I often talk with clients about spiritual disciplines that correspond with their growing psychological edge. For example, a client working on changing their negative thought patterns that contribute to depression and hopelessness may benefit from the daily practice of the prayer of the examen, where they prayerfully review their day to recognize moments of blessing and gratitude. There are many great resources to learn about spiritual disciplines; some of my favorites are noted here.[8]

Flourishing practices. In chapter one, I mentioned a newer branch of psychology called *positive psychology* that focuses on research and interventions to promote human flourishing. Research has demonstrated that positive psychology practices can improve happiness and well-being and contribute to psychological health.[9] Many therapists incorporate positive-psychology practices into the counseling process.

I think one of the most exciting aspects of the positive-psychology movement has been the study of character strengths. By identifying and utilizing our top character strengths in our work and life, we can

[8]Ruth Haley Barton, *Sacred Rhythms: Arranging Our Lives for Spiritual Transformation* (Downers Grove, IL: InterVarsity Press, 2006); Adele Calhoun, *Spiritual Disciplines Handbook: Practices That Transform Us*, 2nd ed. (Downers Grove, IL: InterVarsity Press, 2015).
[9]Alan Carr, Katie Cullen, Cora Keeney, Ciaran Canning, Olwyn Mooney, Ellen Chinseallaigh, and Annie O'Dowd, "Effectiveness of Positive Psychology Interventions: A Systematic Review and Meta-Analysis," *The Journal of Positive Psychology*, 16 no. 6: (2020) 749-69, https://doi.org/10.1080/17439760.2020.1818807

experience a greater sense of meaning, purpose, positive emotion, and achievement. In my work with clients, I have found the research-supported interventions from positive psychology to be quite effective in helping clients develop habits and practices that promote character development. This modern-day application of ancient philosophical and religious understandings of character allows us to connect our deepest values and beliefs with contemporary psychology as we seek to live the good life, not just for ourselves but for the love of God and others.

More Action Steps: Checklist for Creating the Optimal Conditions for Change

Making the most of the counseling experience also involves changing your environment and relationships to support your growth in psychological health and well-being. Interestingly, research on the effectiveness of psychotherapy attributes about 40 percent of the gains made to "extra-therapeutic factors," in other words, the client's environment outside the therapy office.[10] Doing the work of psychotherapy requires clients to create supports in their lives for their new ways of thinking, being, and relating.

Your therapist can help you create the right conditions in your environment for the kind of transformation you hope for. Nothing on this list of five recommendations is rocket science, but it is an encouraging reminder of the holistic nature of the biopsychosocial and spiritual understanding of mental health. Consider one or two recommendations that may be most helpful for you.

Social support. Positive and supportive relationships are necessary for overall mental health and provide important encouragement during the psychotherapy experience. Family, friends, and colleagues can encourage your growth and change, provide feedback, and allow you to try out new relational habits and practices. I often encourage clients to put together a list of people who can be part of a safety net for them as

---

[10]John Norcross and Michael Lambert, "Evidence-Based Therapy Relationships," in *Psychotherapy Relationships That Work: Evidence-Based Responsiveness*, 2nd ed. John Norcross (Oxford: Oxford University Press, 2011), 3-21.

they navigate the ups and downs of the therapy journey and encounter the inevitable challenges. This safety net is quite essential for clients who struggle with self-destructive thoughts or behaviors, and I may make a therapy contract with clients to contact the people on their list for support if they are feeling vulnerable to thoughts of self-harm.

If a client's closest relationships are part of the problem, then a primary goal of therapy will be the development of new sources of social support. One excellent option is to find a support group with others struggling with similar issues who can serve as good travel companions for you during the therapy journey. In support groups, you will connect with others who can normalize difficulties, teach the rules of the road along the way to recovery, and share resources and fruitful practices. A support group also provides an outlet for altruism and caring for others, which is beneficial for your mental health, as you help others even as you are being helped.

Medical check-ups. One of the first questions I ask new clients is when they last had a checkup with their physician, as mental and physical health are closely interrelated. Physicians and mental health professionals regularly work hand in hand to address biopsychosocial problems. When it is difficult to determine the specific etiology of current symptoms, a holistic approach is often warranted to address both physical and psychological symptomatology. Many mental health conditions require a treatment plan that includes both medication and psychotherapy, and clients will want to work with professionals who can coordinate together on treatment goals and interventions.

Physical activity. Adding physical exercise to your routine can provide excellent mental health benefits. Increasing physical activity can contribute greatly to overall brain health and lead to many improvements in mental health and well-being. Most of us, however, have not been very successful at maintaining a healthy exercise routine even though we know the important benefits. Here is where psychological tools such as *behavioral activation* can help jump-start improved habits regarding physical activity. You can implement change strategies toward improving your exercise habits by working with your counselor.

Sleep. Your brain requires good sleep habits to function correctly, and the benefits of therapy can be enhanced by making sure that you are receiving sufficient rest. Improving sleep hygiene is a common goal of counseling, and specific interventions have demonstrated improvement for over 80 percent of clients.[11] If poor sleep is either contributing to your problems or a result of your current struggles, it is of critical importance to raise this issue with your therapist to develop an intervention plan.

Creativity, play, and nature. Just as sleep provides the body and brain with much-needed rest, clients need to include times of creative expression as a respite from the hard work of counseling and psychotherapy. Self-examination can be mind-numbingly arduous, and you will need to ensure that you lift your spirits and lighten your heart through regular doses of life-enhancing activities. For some, finding modes of artistic expression, including art, poetry, and music, provides a valuable adjunct to therapeutic work. Others find that increasing the amount of play and humor in their life provides a helpful balance to the more serious work of psychotherapy. I remember reading about the immunity-boosting effects of laughter during a difficult stage of my own journey and making sure my day included a regular dose of funny animal videos.

One of the lessons many of us learned during the pandemic was the therapeutic and health value of immersing ourselves in nature. Finding moments during the therapy journey to take walks, sit on the front porch, or journal in the park can boost your spirits and provide rest for your body and soul.

Summing Up

I hope the practical guidance offered in this chapter will encourage and empower you to be the primary author of your own story of healing and transformation. You can do much to actively participate in your own

---

[11]Damon K. Ashworth et al., "A Randomized Controlled Trial of Cognitive Behavioral Therapy for Insomnia: An Effective Treatment for Comorbid Insomnia and Depression," *Journal of Counseling Psychology* 62, no. 2 (2015): 115-23, https://doi.org/10.1037/cou000005.9.

healing process through authentic engagement both inside and outside the therapy office. No matter the theoretical approach, counseling sessions can be a transitional, liminal space where you step away from the day-to-day demands of life to be fully present to God and yourself for the essential therapeutic work that can lead to personal transformation. Plus, there are many between-session and environmental strategies you can implement to support the change process.

Take a minute to highlight the action steps from this chapter that stand out to you. What strategies will help you gain the most from your counseling experience? Consider bringing these ideas to your therapist to discuss. And be encouraged—you are now well equipped to bring about the growth and change you most desire.

Roles Recap: Gaining the Most from Counseling

THERAPIST ROLES	CLIENT ROLES
Empower clients to actively participate in and take ownership of their therapy	Take ownership of your therapy experience through active participation in the process
Invite clients to talk about what is most important to them during the therapy hour	Prepare for your counseling sessions by thinking ahead about the issues you want to talk about
Encourage the client's here-and-now processing of deeper needs, feelings, and interpersonal experiences in the session	Be fully present and undistracted during the therapy hour
Provide recommendations for between-session work	Follow through on between-session homework and be curious about obstacles that interfere with completion
Provide education on creating the optimal conditions for growth outside of the counseling office	Make needed changes in your environment to support growth and change

6

Navigating Detours and Impasses Throughout the Counseling Journey

Maybe if I can just avoid thinking about my
problems, they will go away . . .

ME, USING MY DEFAULT (BUT NOT SO HELPFUL)
COPING STRATEGY

All journeys involve the unexpected, and the counseling journey is no exception. Detours, impasses, and roadblocks are inevitable in the growth process. This chapter will identify the common supports and barriers you can expect on the road to mental health. We will look more closely at the change process and outline specific actions that clients and therapists can take to keep growth in therapy moving forward. We will identify common challenges and how to navigate in, around, or through them.

The middle phase of therapy can be the most challenging part of the journey as you delve deeper into the problematic thoughts, feelings, and behaviors that you may have been sidestepping for a long time. It is common during this phase for clients to feel more discomfort and distress as they face truths about themselves they would rather avoid. Many people feel ambivalent about giving up old and familiar ways of thought and action as they count the cost of making fundamental changes in their lives. At this stage in the journey, it may be tempting to think about calling it a day, heading home, and giving up on the counseling journey altogether.

But it is imperative at this stage that you do not lose hope. These challenges are a normal part of the therapeutic process and often indicate that you are really getting somewhere in your work. What appears to be an impasse frequently becomes the very opportunity needed to further your growth and development. You can draw on many supports and strategies to help you run the race with endurance toward your therapeutic goals.

How Do I Know IF I Am Making Progress?

The question on most clients' minds in the middle phase of therapy is this: "Am I making progress?" Psychotherapy is a significant investment of time and resources, and it is crucial to be able to have confidence that you are moving in the right direction and making positive gains. The challenge in tracking progress is that therapy is often a nonlinear journey. At times, it can feel like you are going in circles, returning to the same issues repeatedly. This is actually an important part of the process, as you have the opportunity for deeper exploration and new insights each time you revisit the same issues. But how do you measure overall progress?

Assessing progress is a collaborative endeavor between the client and therapist where we review treatment goals, recognize areas of improvement, and identify the issues that require further attention. Through collaborative assessment, we fine-tune your goals and adjust the treatment plan as needed.

Signs of progress in therapy may include any of the following:

- a decrease in negative or distressing thoughts and feelings
- increased self-awareness and insight into issues, patterns, and needs
- improvements in relationships
- greater capacity for coping with stressful life events
- improved regulation of emotions, including greater emotional awareness and acceptance
- changes and improvements in targeted behaviors
- decreased sense of isolation
- clearer sense of identity, meaning, and purpose

- growth in faith and spiritual maturity
- greater self-compassion and acceptance

Therapists invite feedback from clients on how the process of counseling is going, what has been helpful, and what needs to change for the experience to be most useful and effective. This may include asking clients to complete symptom checklists or brief outcome assessment scales at the end of sessions to track progress. As therapists, we have an ethical commitment to ensure that the services we provide are helpful to our clients, and we depend on our clients' honest input to ensure that we are providing the best possible treatment. As clients, it is important to provide honest feedback about the therapy experience so that an accurate assessment of progress can occur. Clients must voice their concerns about the therapeutic process with their counselor. Rather than hurting the counselor's feelings or offending them, honest feedback indicates that a productive and resilient psychotherapy relationship is developing. Later in the chapter, we will explore specific strategies for how you can raise your concerns with your counselor to address any barriers to the counseling process.

How Do People Change?

Understanding the process involved in change can be quite helpful for clients and therapists so we can identify together where the process might be stuck and how to move forward. Social scientists have studied the science of human behavioral change for many years, and we now know quite a bit about the mechanisms and processes involved. This line of research has had many important implications for helping people make healthy lifestyle adjustments.

One of the most widely regarded change theories is the *Transtheoretical Model of Change*, sometimes called the *stages of change*.[1] Developed by James Prochaska and Carlo DiClemente in the late 1970s, the

---

[1]James O. Prochaska, Carlo C. DiClemente, and John C. Norcross, "In Search of How People Change: Applications to Addictive Behaviors," *American Psychologist* 47, no. 9 (1992): 1102-14, doi:10.1037//0003-066x.47.9.1102.

stages of change describe the typical phases people go through in changing behavior and identify essential processes that can keep us moving forward. Research over the past twenty-five years has explored the application of this model to health issues, including medication compliance, weight loss, smoking cessation, anxiety, and depression. Let's briefly look at the six stages of change and strategies for advancing the change process.[2]

Precontemplation. At this stage clients are not yet committed to change. If problem behavior is brought to their attention, they may say, "I'll work on that issue in the future." Clients in the precontemplation stage of change are probably in counseling at someone else's insistence. They may view the problem as other people and not themselves. They may not necessarily be resistant to change but may have tried in the past and failed, and thus feel demoralized or unable to change. At the precontemplation stage of change, a client might say something like this: "My employer requires me to get some counseling to improve my teamwork skills. I work with some difficult people, and we have had a lot of conflict. I am not sure what counseling can do to help the situation."

At this stage, the cons of changing are much greater than the pros. You can move toward change by increasing the pro side of the list and considering the benefits of change as well as the consequences of not changing. It may also be helpful to conduct an honest assessment of the problem's impact on yourself and others.

Contemplation. In this stage, the pros and cons of change are more equal, and people are seriously weighing the costs of embarking on the change process. A client at this stage of change may feel a sense of ambivalence about giving up or changing certain behaviors and continue to consider the costs and benefits. They may struggle with a sense of "Can I really do this?" Focusing on the positive benefits of change is an important strategy at this stage. A client in the contemplation stage might say, "I know I am an opinionated person, and it offends some people on

[2]James O. Prochaska, "Transtheoretical Model of Behavior Change," in *Encyclopedia of Behavioral Medicine*, ed. Marc D. Gellman and J. Rick Turner (New York: Springer, 2013): 1997-2000.

my team when I push hard to get my point across. But I also want good relationships at work and could probably do better at listening."

Planning. People in the planning stage have decided to embark on a process of change and need a solid plan of action. They may be worried about failing and wonder whether they can be successful. Clients at this stage need encouragement, confidence boosting, and help with proven strategies for changing specific behaviors.

Our client struggling with relationships at work might say something like this in the planning stage: "We have been talking about my relationships at work, but I think I can also be insensitive in my relationships with family and friends. Maybe this is a problem I need to work on. How can counseling help me with this?"

Action. The most active phase of the change process, the action stage, involves the client's focused and engaged actions toward changing behaviors with tangible results. Clients may begin to experience the benefits of change that may positively alter their views of themselves. They are involved in working hard to resist relapse and keep moving forward with behavioral changes. At this stage, successful change processes include improving self-efficacy (or the confidence that you *can* change), support from others, and rewarding positive change behaviors.

Maintenance. Once positive behavioral changes are made, clients must also learn to maintain them long-term. The main task of maintenance is preventing relapse through changing the environments, recognizing triggers, and seeking the ongoing support that is needed to sustain change. Clients learn to incorporate healthy substitutes for problem behaviors, for example, calling a friend for support rather than isolating or avoiding social situations.

Termination. While many people stay in the maintenance stage indefinitely, Prochaska estimates that about 20 percent can progress to a termination phase of change, where there is complete confidence that the change is permanent with minimal risk of relapse.[3] Rather than a linear progression through these six stages, the change process for many

---

[3]Prochaska, "Transtheoretical Model of Behavioral Change."

people looks more like a spiral of relapse and then recovery, learning from your lapses to strengthen your resolve, and reengaging with your strategies for change.

Specific change strategies. Prochaska and colleagues identify many strategies to help people move forward in the change process.[4]

- Commit to change and believe that you can be successful.
- Conduct an honest assessment of the impact of problem behaviors on your life and others.
- List the pros and cons of change and seek to add to the pro side of the equation.
- Enlist expert guidance for the change process—a therapist or coach.
- Surround yourself with others who are also involved in changing similar behaviors.
- Identify triggers in your environment for the problem behavior.
- Improve your environment by strengthening supports and minimizing triggers.
- Substitute the unhealthy behavior with a healthy practice.
- Reward yourself for reaching milestones.
- Rewrite your self-scripts to focus on empowering and encouraging self-statements to increase self-efficacy.

As we wrap up this review of the psychology of change, I invite you to take a moment to identify where you are right now in the process of change. What would it take to move one step closer to the next stage? Consider highlighting one or two specific action steps on the checklist above and plan how to implement this step in the upcoming week. Share your commitment with a supportive friend, family member, or your therapist. Review your progress in a week and celebrate each small step you have achieved. You are taking an invaluable step in the change process even by completing this simple exercise—well done!

---

[4]Prochaska, DiClemente, and Norcross, "In Search of How People Change."

Embracing Both Acceptance and Change in Psychotherapy

While it may seem paradoxical, one aspect of change is the *acceptance* that some aspects of yourself may not be changeable. We all face biological, psychological, relational, or environmental challenges that may be enduring. We learn to live with our histories, past mistakes, and memories of difficult experiences. Psychotherapy can lessen the negative psychological impact of these conditions while also increasing your capacity for acceptance of enduring conditions. Through counseling, you can identify when acceptance is, paradoxically, the best course of action.

You will likely realize at some point during your personal growth journey that there are aspects of your personality and experiences that you will carry with you indefinitely. You may have made much progress in dealing with problematic thoughts, feelings, and behaviors so your symptoms no longer interfere with your daily life. But you may need to accept that you will continue to live with your vulnerability to these symptoms as you recognize potential triggers that remind you to use your good coping skills.

Ongoing challenges can remind us that we are part of a common humanity and are not immune to life's difficulties. Our acceptance of enduring issues keeps us humble, compassionate, and deeply aware of our need for others to support our continued growth and development.

A common example of the importance of acceptance is when clients are diagnosed with a chronic medical or psychiatric condition. As discussed earlier in the book, many clients feel relieved when they realize that their symptoms constitute a diagnosable condition. However, it can be daunting to recognize that the condition may require a long-term commitment to a course of treatment. Focusing only on change rather than acceptance of a chronic condition can actually impede progress and potentially foster denial. I see this often when clients are diagnosed with a chronic or severe mental illness that requires a long-term commitment to a treatment plan that may include medication, psychotherapy, and social support for the person to function adaptively. A lack of acceptance of a chronic mental illness can lead to inconsistent engagement with treatment, which will impede the client's return to more stable functioning and cause more ongoing difficulties for the client and their family.

For acceptance work with clients, I appreciate the approach to psychotherapy called acceptance and commitment therapy.[5] Acceptance and commitment therapy helps clients focus less on getting rid of unwanted symptoms and more on moving forward in life in the direction of values and commitments regardless of their symptoms. Using interventions and strategies, clients can learn to be present in their day-to-day lives, curious and aware of ongoing symptoms, but allowing their deeply held values and commitments to take center stage in guiding actions and decisions. In other words, acceptance and commitment therapy can provide strategies to change clients' relationship with those thoughts, feelings, and experiences that they may carry with them indefinitely, accepting their presence and gaining distance from them while moving forward with living a purposeful life.

I can think of many clients over the years who have made significant progress in dealing with complex and traumatic experiences. While they have experienced substantial healing and growth, they also realize that their histories will always be a part of their story, albeit with less harmful impact. They have engaged in the hard work of transforming their life story to one of survival, strength, and hope (change work) while also recognizing the very real adverse experiences that have occurred in their lives (acceptance work), weaving acceptance and change into their life narrative in meaningful and empowering ways. One client described the outcome in this way: "I need to remember where I have been as it helps me connect with others who are facing similar difficulties."

Accepting a chronic condition or unwanted aspects of yourself can be difficult. It helps tremendously to have the guidance and support of a therapist to help discern where in your life to focus on change, and which areas may require greater acceptance.

---

[5]Steven C. Hayes, *Get Out of Your Mind and into Your Life* (Oakland, CA: New Harbinger, 2005).

Common Roadblocks, Detours, and Impasses to Change (and What Can Be Done About Them)

Another paradoxical challenge we have learned about the human condition is that we all develop self-protective coping strategies to help us deal with stressful, difficult, and anxiety-inducing life circumstances. Coping behaviors can be positive and adaptive, such as learning to recognize danger and remove ourselves from potential threats, or using deep breathing to stay calm in stressful situations. Coping strategies can also be negative and lead to further problems, such as using drugs or alcohol to numb painful feelings.[6] At times, we may be aware of our positive and negative coping strategies while they are happening. But they can also occur automatically and outside our awareness.

As people grow and develop, some of the same protective coping tactics that provided protection earlier in life can become harmful and limit the ability to deal with life circumstances effectively. Take, for example, the child who learned early on in life to escape the painful reality of his parents' constant fighting in the home by retreating into a fantasy world through video games, books, and movies. This coping skill can become problematic during his adult life if he cannot productively work through interpersonal conflicts in the workplace, for example, and escapes into fantasy by playing video games at his desk. These potential roadblocks to change can be psychological, behavioral, and cognitive.[7] Let's look at some common examples of each.

Psychological roadblocks. Psychological resistance to change is often based on conscious and unconscious fears clients have about whether their lives will improve if they risk doing things differently. A client may struggle with perfectionistic tendencies and worry about making mistakes if they try to change. Or some may prefer to live their lives in a highly structured, predictable manner that avoids risks and seeks

---

[6]"Coping behavior," APA Dictionary of Psychology, April 19, 2018, https://dictionary.apa .org/coping-behavior.
[7]Lena Forsell and Jan A. Åström, "An Analysis of Resistance to Change Exposed in Individuals' Thoughts and Behaviors," *Comprehensive Psychology* 1 (2012), https://doi.org /10.2466/09.02.10.CP.1.17.

familiar routines. Familiar dysfunction can feel safer than new ways of thinking and behaving, thus keeping clients stuck. These psychological protective strategies are called *defense mechanisms*. Defense mechanisms are the automatic and sometimes unconscious coping strategies people have used throughout life to protect them from perceived threats and change. The defense mechanisms we use over time can become part of our personality style and impact the way we relate to others.

Common psychological defense mechanisms that come up in therapy can include:

- *avoidance* coping strategies, which include ways of thinking and behaving that allow clients to dodge the real issues that may be difficult to deal with
- *denial* strategies, where clients refute or reject admission of their current struggles, symptoms, or behaviors
- *intellectualization*, whereby clients try to reason away their current emotional struggles to avoid painful feelings
- *rationalization*, which occurs when clients try to justify problematic thoughts, feelings, or behaviors
- *externalization*, blaming others or external circumstances for one's own actions and behaviors
- *somatization*, the development of physiological symptoms as a result of unacknowledged psychological distress
- *projection*, which occurs when clients see their own psychological issues, fears, and anxiety in others that they are not able to acknowledge in themselves
- *emotional numbing*, when clients try to cope with difficult feelings through addictive behaviors such as drugs, alcohol, food, gambling, and workaholic tendencies

Do any of these protective strategies sound familiar to you? If so, you are in good company. We all fall back on psychological defense mechanisms in times of uncertainty and change. Identifying and naming your psychological barriers to change are essential steps toward getting unstuck in your personal growth and development process.

Secondary gain and learned helplessness. A behavioral perspective on obstacles to change invites clients to look at how their current environment, including their relationships, may reinforce or maintain their current symptoms. Secondary gain involves the hidden advantages of having a physical or mental illness and the anticipated losses that would occur if the symptoms were to resolve. It is worth considering whether there are secondary gains for maintaining the status quo that may even be operating unconsciously. For example, an adolescent or young adult from a conflictual or disengaged family may learn that it takes a crisis or failure on their part for the family to come together in unity and support. Thus, a secondary gain exists for remaining in perpetual turmoil and dysfunction. It is important to note that secondary gain often operates outside our awareness and may require the help of others to identify.

An additional way the environment can contribute to barriers to change is the phenomenon of learned helplessness, where clients have tried repeatedly to change an issue without success, resulting in a sense of helpless despair. Common to clients with depression, learned helplessness can be ameliorated through strategies such as behavioral activation or competency shaping, where clients are encouraged to take small, successful steps toward a desired outcome and recognize their progress in the right direction. For example, I might encourage a client struggling to get on a program of regular physical exercise to take a walk around their neighborhood block once a day rather than pay for an expensive gym membership and affirm the small step they are taking toward their goal of improved physical fitness.

Cognitive barriers to change. Frequently, in therapeutic work, clients will become aware of irrational beliefs and unrealistic expectations that are like giant boulders impeding their pathway to growth and development. One client, for example, believed that she could not try new ways of thinking and acting unless she could do it perfectly the first time. Another client thought he did not deserve to be happy when others in his family of origin were still stuck in dysfunctional patterns and addictions. Other clients may be so sure they will fail that the barriers to change feel insurmountable. Through the counseling process, we can track these negative thinking patterns, identify the irrational core beliefs that the thoughts originate from, and take steps to replace them with more accurate views of self, others, and the world.

Dealing with your defense mechanisms. Take a moment to review these examples of common barriers to change. Which ones resonate with you? Remember that these coping strategies probably served a protective function at some point in your life when they were most needed to keep you from psychological harm. But now, they are most likely keeping you from a healthier way of thinking, feeling, and doing. It is time to trade them in for more adaptive ways of dealing with life's difficulties.

As counselors, we will work with you to bring these unconscious, sometimes self-sabotaging, defense mechanisms into conscious awareness to be examined and understood. We will help you assess where you are in the process of change and facilitate your forward movement by providing support, challenges, opportunities for honest assessment of pros and cons, and action strategies. We will help you move toward acceptance of enduring challenges that may not be changeable.

One common strategy therapists use to help facilitate change is to ask clients to envision their desired outcomes with great specificity. This can include homework assignments where clients write about their ideal life, vocation, and relationships. A popular intervention is called the *miracle question*, where we ask clients, If you were to wake up tomorrow and your problems were gone, how would you know? What would your life look like? Describing specific markers of growth and progress can help you recognize them when they occur.

We can also prescribe to clients that they engage in some of the very behaviors they feel helpless to avoid (this does not include self-destructive or harmful behaviors, such as prescribing substance abuse, for example). For a client who cannot stop worrying about a specific issue, I may ask them to schedule a daily *worry time* where they save up all of their anxious thoughts and spend an hour thinking about their concerns. This assignment fosters the realization that dwelling on anxious thoughts is something they can exert more control over, leading to a greater sense of self-efficacy and decreased helplessness.

As therapists, we have many strategies for addressing psychological defenses that can impede change. Together, you and your therapist can identify the inevitable barriers to change and implement interventions to keep the process of growth and development moving forward.

Dealing with Impasses in the Therapeutic Relationship

A friend recently shared her ambivalence about her current therapy experience, describing her uncertainly about whether it was helpful. "Is the problem me or my therapist?" she wondered. In the end, she decided to discontinue her counseling and confessed that she opted to disappear rather than talk with her therapist about how she was feeling. "I was afraid to hurt my therapist's feelings," she acknowledged.

Questions and difficulties in the therapeutic relationship are an inevitable and essential part of counseling. Called *impasses*, these bumpy moments in the counseling process can feel like roadblocks that keep us from moving forward. Often they reflect the interpersonal challenges clients experience with other people in their lives and can provide tremendous insight into the similar relational barriers that keep them from becoming the people they most want to be. However, impasses in the therapeutic relationship can feel difficult to navigate and may create a sense of doubt for clients in themselves (Am I a lousy client?), their therapist (Maybe I have a lousy therapist?), and in the therapeutic process (Maybe therapy doesn't work for me?).

When these questions inevitably occur, I encourage you to summon your courage and raise your concerns with your therapist. Therapists can help this process by making time in sessions to evaluate progress or inviting clients to talk openly about fears, frustrations, and unmet expectations. Telling your counselor you are frustrated with them for some action on their part will likely bring greater benefit to your personal growth journey than quitting therapy to avoid having a difficult conversation.

Too often, I have seen people drop out of therapy because of an impasse right at the time they are poised for a breakthrough. If I could offer advice from my forty years of experience as a therapist, it would be this:

don't run, avoid, or escape from therapeutic impasses. Embrace them as opportunities for change. More often than not, impasses will open up the pathway to change that you have been hoping for all along. How can this be?

Enactments. We have previously considered how the difficulties in the therapy relationship may mirror some of the challenges you experience in other relationships. It is unsurprising that as therapy progresses, fears, feelings, and unmet expectations emerge in the counseling relationship, similar to other relationships. Rather than hindering the therapy process, these *enactments* provide a valuable window for the client and therapist to examine the interpersonal patterns together as what happens outside the therapy room is brought within. The immediacy of working with the here-and-now relationship in therapy can be initially anxiety-producing, but in the end, it can be one of the most effective and impactful therapeutic opportunities for real change. In other words, the therapeutic relationship can provide a corrective emotional experience to past relational injuries. The benefits from this corrective experience can then be generalized to other relationships in clients' lives.

Let me give you an example from my own experience as a client during my graduate school years. My psychologist had been helping me gain insights into my difficulties with vulnerability and asking others for help, which had led to an unhealthy self-sufficiency based on my belief that significant others would not be there for me when I most needed them. The following week, I showed up for what I thought was our next appointment, only to realize after half an hour in the waiting room that I had "forgotten" that my therapist was on vacation that week. I left the office in tears with that familiar feeling that I could not rely on anyone, including my therapist. We processed this experience the following week in session, and I recognized that I had re-created a relational pattern that reinforced my belief that if I am vulnerable, significant others will not be there for me. This enactment was a pivotal moment in our treatment of gaining insight into my interactional patterns with others.

It is essential to acknowledge that as therapists, we bring our own issues to the counseling experience, too, that contribute to the enactments of our own interpersonal patterns. Fortunately, one of our job requirements is *reflective practice*, which requires us to dig into our own issues that can get stirred up by our counseling work. We seek out regular consultation with peers and supervisors as well as our own therapy to ensure that our work with clients is not adversely affected by what is going on in our personal lives and that we are not oversharing our struggles. Interestingly, I have found that I do some of my best counseling work with clients when I am also in a place of suffering and struggle in my personal life. I can only surmise that times of personal difficulty help me be especially attuned to the suffering of my clients more deeply and intuitively.

Rupture and repair of the therapeutic relationship. Moments of disconnection, disappointment, and unmet expectations are an inevitable part of the therapy process, and it is important that these experiences are identified and expressed. Often, clients hesitate to bring up their frustrations with the therapist out of concern that the therapist will be hurt, angry, or even blame the client for the problems. Clients can also assume that if therapy is not going well, they must be the problem, thus they avoid expressing their needs and concerns about the process. However, you will gain the most from the therapy experience when you voice both your positive and negative relational experiences with the counselor.

As therapists, we work very hard to provide you with a professional, reliable, consistent, and safe counseling experience. But we are also very human and will inevitably do our job imperfectly, come late to sessions, forget important information, and say unhelpful things (or stay silent when you need us to say something!). We may miss important cues from you that a relational rupture has occurred. We need your help knowing when something is going on in the therapeutic relationship that is affecting your ability to trust us so we can repair the relationship and restore your confidence in us and the therapy process.

I recall one client who came into therapy quite upset about our previous session, where we had talked in depth about his harrowing experiences serving in the military during the Gulf War. It was the first time he shared these experiences with me, and I felt we had made good progress in the session. However, he reported that he left the session flooded with memories and experiences that were disturbing to him throughout the week. He felt I had allowed him to share too much too soon and wished I had slowed the process the previous week. We were able to repair this rupture in our relationship as I acknowledged that I missed the cues that he was upset during the session and did not realize he had left in a state of distress. We had a productive session about how to pace our sessions better, ensuring that we spent some time at the end of each session helping him contain distressing memories, and also agreed to do more work on coping strategies he could use between sessions. We recognized that this experience was an enactment for him of many other relational experiences where he felt unprotected by people he put his trust in—parents, military supervisors, and now his therapist. The rupture-and-repair experience provided him with a blueprint for how honest sharing of his needs and experiences could enact change in his important relationships. In short, his courageous initiative to share his feelings with me yielded some important therapeutic work for him, as well as invaluable personal and professional insights for me about the importance of pacing and timing in my work with traumatized clients.

So, how do you address your questions, frustrations, and disappointments about the counseling process with your therapist? Here are some possible conversation starters:

- I have some questions about our counseling work—can we take some time today to discuss them?
- I appreciate the work we have been doing in counseling, but I am concerned that I am not seeing the improvements I hoped for. Can we take some time today to evaluate my progress?
- I expected I would receive more (or less) of _____ from therapy.
- I would like to talk about what happened during the last session. I felt _____ when _____.

- It is helpful to me when _____ happens in our sessions.
- It is not helpful to me when _____ happens in our sessions.
- I feel like we are coming at this issue from different perspectives, and I am not sure you understand _____ about my experience.

Remember, as therapists, we need your help letting us know when we are encountering a relational impasse or rupture that needs repair. While it can feel awkward to bring up issues about the therapeutic relationship, it is an important and necessary part of the process.

When a therapeutic impasse becomes a roadblock. Sometimes, impasses in therapy become roadblocks that cannot successfully be addressed, even when we make our best effort. It is absolutely your right as a client to find another counselor if your current therapist is not the best fit for you. How do you know when to stay with your current therapist and work through impasses versus moving on to another counselor? Here are some signs that it may be time to find a new therapist:

- ongoing lack of progress toward your therapy goals, even after you've given it some time
- your attempts to raise concerns about your progress or questions about counseling are met with defensiveness or resistance from the counselor
- you do not feel a sense of trust and connection with your therapist
- you feel your therapist does not understand and/or respect important aspects of who you are, for example, your age, gender, race and ethnicity, differential abilities, religion, etc.
- your therapist does not seem to have sufficient expertise or experience with your presenting issues
- Most importantly, unethical behaviors on the part of your therapist, including a breach of confidentiality, boundary violation, or discriminatory behavior, are a sure sign for you to find another counselor. As discussed in chapter three, professional ethics are foundational to the safety and effectiveness of the counseling experience and provide necessary protection for clients. You can file

an ethics complaint with your state licensing board if your therapist acts unethically.

Ideally, speaking with your counselor about your decision to find a new therapist is beneficial and helps to bring closure to your therapy experience, even if the work is unfinished. Counselors have an ethical duty to refer clients to another provider if the client is not improving or receiving benefits from treatment. If this occurs, your counselor should provide you with the names of several qualified therapists.

While it can be challenging to change therapists, I believe all therapeutic encounters move us forward toward health and healing, even if we have to change lanes to find a new guide who may be a better fit for our needs. What is important is that you do not give up on your counseling journey but rather find a better path to travel further toward your goals.

Faith Perspectives: Religious and Spiritual Supports and Challenges

Many clients find that their religious beliefs and practices can be transformative during the counseling journey. Over the past twenty years, there has been growing scientific evidence supporting the use of religious and spiritual practices to benefit people's mental health.[8] Individual and community spiritual practices can help us cope with life's difficulties, give meaning to experiences of suffering, and guide us in living our most full and meaningful lives.[9] Growth in spiritual maturity and psychological health can go hand in hand as spiritual practices boost the effectiveness of psychological interventions. As discussed throughout this book, clients and counselors can work together to incorporate spiritual practices into the psychotherapy process.[10]

---

[8]Harold G. Koenig, "Religion, Spirituality, and Health: The Research and Clinical Implications," *ISRN Psychiatry*, December 16, 2012, 10-23, doi:10.5402/2012/278730.

[9]Koenig, "Religion, Spirituality, and Health," 23-26.

[10]For examples of integration of Christian practices with positive psychology, see Terri Watson, "Living Well in Christ: Practical Wisdom from Positive Psychology," Tower Talks at Wheaton College, May 9, 2019, 15:24, www.youtube.com/watch?v=BTJxkpSMzFY.

Studies of religious coping have discovered that people tend to use their religious views in both positive and negative ways during experiences of adversity.[11] People who use positive religious coping tend to experience a strong sense of closeness to God and others in their religious communities during times of suffering. They view God as directing, empowering, and leading their efforts to cope. With negative religious coping, people tend to feel disconnected from God and others during stressful life events and may even feel their suffering is a punishment from God. Negative religious coping can be a barrier to mental health for clients when it fosters inaccurate views of God, themselves self, and their suffering.

Religious and spiritual attitudes can be a hindrance to growth and development when people overly spiritualize mental health treatment or misuse spiritual practices to avoid the hard work of dealing with painful experiences. The term *spiritual bypass* refers to the use of spirituality as a psychological defense to shortcut, avoid, or take a detour around necessary personal or relational growth.[12] A client who is struggling with an addiction may assert, for example, that they do not need to seek treatment or attend Alcoholics Anonymous because they can gain all the help they need through prayer. A client diagnosed with a severe mental illness may refuse medication in the belief that God will heal them if they have faith. Indeed, God can and does heal people from disease, but most often it requires active work through engagement in the available treatment options.

Recognizing negative spiritual coping and spiritual bypass as barriers to growth and development does not negate the importance and validity of healthy spiritual practices, which can be incorporated into the counseling process. The journey toward health and wholeness often requires steady and courageous progress *through* our pain. It is human nature to

---

[11]Kenneth I. Pargament et al., "The Religious Dimensions of Coping: Advances in Theory, Research, and Practice," in *Handbook of the Psychology of Religion and Spirituality*, 2nd ed., ed. Raymond Paloutzian and Crystal Park (New York: Guilford, 2013), 560-79.

[12]Gabriela Picciotto, Jesse Fox, and Félix Neto, "A Phenomenology of Spiritual Bypass: Causes, Consequences, and Implications," *Journal of Spirituality in Mental Health* (2017), doi:10.1080/19349637.2017.1417756.

want to find detours and shortcuts to avoid the hard work of therapy. These detours will often manifest in client's use of defense mechanisms and lead them down a dead end where they will have to backtrack and eventually do the hard work of growth through suffering. How do you know whether you are using spiritual practices to promote spiritual and psychological health, versus engaging in spiritual bypassing? This is a thoughtful question for discernment that you may not be able to answer for yourself without the help of a therapist, spiritual adviser, or wise spiritual friend.

I deeply appreciate faithful men and women throughout history who have articulated through their writings the rhythms of the spiritual journey, which include times of consolation and desolation, growth and stagnation, and nearness to God followed by dark nights of the soul. In the Psalms, for example, David pours out his lament in these words:

> LORD, do not rebuke me in your anger
>> or discipline me in your wrath.
> Have mercy on me, LORD, for I am faint;
>> heal me, LORD, for my bones are in agony.
> My soul is in deep anguish.
>> How long, LORD, how long?
> Turn, LORD, and deliver me;
>> save me because of your unfailing love. (Psalm 6:1-4)

When we need courageous endurance of suffering, it can be *en-couraging* to read the stories of the great cloud of witnesses who have gone before us. We can draw strength from the exemplars in our faith traditions who experienced great adversity in pursuing God's call, even to the point of death, with Jesus as the ultimate example. As Hebrews 12:3 says, "Consider him who endured such opposition from sinners, so that you will not grow weary and lose heart."

Action Step: Self-Assessment of Supports and Challenges

As we reach the end of the chapter, I encourage you to take some time to reflect on the supports and challenges that may affect your own personal growth journey. Consider the following questions for self-reflection:

- Where do I see progress or improvement in my mental health journey?
- Where do I feel stuck?
- Which of the stages of change best describes my current experience?
- What change strategies can I try this week?
- What areas of my life and experience may require greater acceptance and less of a focus on change?
- Which of the psychological, behavioral, and cognitive defensive or coping strategies do I tend to rely on?
- What are the relational patterns I enact in my interactions with others, and how do they signal areas that need healing?
- How do my spiritual beliefs and practices provide growth and support during adversity and suffering?
- Where do I recognize the risk of negative spiritual coping or spiritual bypass as a barrier to psychological and spiritual maturity?

We all have familiar attitudes and behaviors that can hijack our growth and development. What is important is that you find the strength to courageously self-assess how you get in your own way. You are taking a significant step in your own process of change by considering the supports and challenges described in this chapter and how they might apply to you.

Summing Up

Over the years of conducting psychotherapy, I have observed a certain rhythm to the counseling journey. The first phase of therapy is often quite rewarding, as clients are able to name their current difficulties, develop insight into how the problems occurred, and implement effective coping skills that lead to symptom relief and self-improvement. Then we enter the middle phase of therapy, where clients begin to touch on some of the deeper and more vulnerable issues that lie behind problematic behaviors, thoughts, and feelings. Inevitably, the self-protective defense mechanisms kick in, and clients can encounter what can feel like impasses, detours, and slowdowns. The middle stage of therapy is, in many ways, the *working-through* stage, where clients have the opportunity to address the same barriers to health and change that they encounter in their day-to-day lives.

This is a critical time in the counseling journey when you may become discouraged and consider discontinuing treatment. I hope you are encouraged to know that this is a normal and expected part of the process of growth and change. There are many ways that you and your therapist can turn these impasses into critical moments of insight and growth.

We can then move to the last stage of therapy, the *carrying-forward* stage, where you and your therapist will apply your new insights to old problems and prepare you to continue the mental health journey on your own. This last phase is the topic for our next chapter.

Roles Recap: Navigating Detours and Impasses

THERAPIST ROLES	CLIENT ROLES
Invite regular feedback about the client's experience of counseling	Provide honest feedback and voice questions and concerns
Initiate collaborative assessment of progress	Accurately report changes in symptoms and problems
Implement both change and acceptance interventions as appropriate	Implement both change and acceptance interventions as appropriate
Assess coping and defense mechanisms and help the client address the barriers to change	Understand the protective role of defense mechanisms and try out new and healthier coping strategies
Raise here-and-now conversations about the therapeutic relationship and initiate the repair of ruptures; acknowledge therapist mistakes!	Voice concerns with the therapeutic relationship as opportunities for relational growth
Identify spiritual and religious supports and barriers to the process of growth and change	Explore positive and negative religious coping strategies and draw from spiritual practices to promote healthy spiritual and psychological growth

7

Ending Well

Are we there yet?

ACCORDING TO URBAN DICTIONARY, "A PHRASE
USED BY PASSENGERS TRAPPED IN A VEHICLE
FOR ANY PERIOD OF TIME. ORIGINATES
IN CHILDHOOD AND EXTENDS TO ROAD TRIPS"

"Are we there yet?" is perhaps the universal question on the minds of travelers as we near the ends of our journeys, whether road trips, hikes, pilgrimages, or in this case the counseling journey. For clients, the question "How do I know when I am finished with therapy?" can feel both exciting and anxiety-producing. When approached thoughtfully and intentionally, the last stage of therapy can be an encouraging and affirming process that provides an opportunity to consolidate gains made in treatment, anticipate setbacks, and end well.

However, endings also activate our prior losses and inadequately processed grief. It is tempting for clients to want to avoid this last stage of therapy by prematurely terminating their treatment, canceling sessions, or not showing up for appointments. It is estimated that one out of five clients will drop out of therapy prematurely and as a result may experience fewer overall benefits from psychotherapy.[1]

In this chapter we will look at the last phase of the counseling journey as a positive opportunity to both end *well* and *end* well. Ending *well* involves recognizing and embracing your gains in therapy as you transition with hope and confidence from the counseling journey to a lifelong adventure

---

[1]Joshua K. Swift and Roger P. Greenberg, "Premature Discontinuation in Adult Psychotherapy: A Meta-Analysis," *Journal of Consulting and Clinical Psychology* 80, no. 4 (2012): 547-59, doi:10.1037/a0028226.

of continued personal growth and health. *Ending* well affirms the excellent work you and your counselor have accomplished together, brings closure to your relationship, and provides the confidence you will need to enact the changes made in the counseling office into your day-to-day life.

How Do I Know When I Am Ready to End Therapy?

Theresa and I had been meeting together for about six months. When she began therapy, she was experiencing significant distress, and our weekly time barely seemed enough to process the stressors in her life, work on coping skills, and make sense of the difficulties she was having in relationships. However, for the past month, Theresa reported improvements in her mood, relationships, and confidence in her ability to cope. She used our session time more for reporting on the week's events with less of a need to process or problem-solve the difficulties in her life. After I made this observation, we revisited her goals for psychotherapy and recognized the progress she had made toward meeting them. Together, we began to talk about whether it was time to bring our counseling work to a close.

The decision to end therapy is a mutual and collaborative process between the client and therapist. It involves evaluating the progress made and assessing the client's readiness to continue their mental health journey outside therapy. I have found six signposts that signal that the counseling work may be nearing an end:

1. The client has gained self-awareness of their problems, how they developed, and how to cope with them in the future.

2. The client is functioning well at home, work or school, and in their relationships.

3. The gains made in counseling have been generalized or applied to the client's day-to-day life.

4. There is an improvement in coping skills in response to life stressors.

5. The client is showing greater emotional awareness and the ability to regulate their emotions.

6. The client demonstrates increasing confidence in managing problems and navigating setbacks.

Ending *well* involves recognizing signs of increased well-being and improved mental health to signal that therapy is nearing the end. To revisit our definition of wellness from chapter one: "a state of mental well-being that enables people to cope with the stresses of life, to realize their abilities, to learn well and work well, and to contribute to their communities."[2]

How long is the end phase of the counseling journey? Ending psychotherapy is a process and may require several sessions to bring the work to closure. The length of time devoted to the ending process must be customized for each client and therapist and is affected by the length of the course of therapy. For a client whom I have seen for a few months, one or two sessions of bringing our work to a close should suffice. Clients who have been in therapy for a more extended period of time will benefit from a longer process to consolidate the gains made and bring closure to the therapy relationship. Clients with a significant loss history will require careful attention to the ending process to provide a corrective emotional experience compared to other unresolved losses.

Sometimes clients express a desire to continue counseling primarily for support. When this is the case, we assess together whether there are other, more natural sources of support that the client can cultivate or utilize. We may decrease sessions to once per month for maintenance or supportive sessions. I even have clients who schedule an annual checkup with me to address any issues that come up and ensure that they are staying on course with their mental health goals.

Not all psychotherapy endings occur because the work is finished, however. Life happens, and sometimes people move, insurance coverage changes, or clients find it challenging to carve out the time for therapy in the busyness of life. Sometimes there is a recognition of a lack of goodness of fit between client and therapist, or a therapeutic alliance does not form. There may be insufficient progress in therapy. If this is the case, the counselor has an ethical commitment to discontinue the counseling if it no longer benefits the client and to provide referrals to

---

[2]"World Mental Health Report: Transforming Mental Health for All," World Health Organization, 2022, 8, www.who.int/publications/i/item/9789240049338.

other qualified professionals. It is still important in these circumstances to take time to review the work that has been accomplished and bring some closure to the counseling experience. I make it a point to assure clients that the door is always open if they should choose to pursue therapy again in the future.

The End Stage of the Counseling Journey: Essential Tasks

Research on the end stage of psychotherapy has found that a large majority of clients experience the end of treatment as a positive experience and a catalyst for continued growth and positive mental health.[3] Even clients with significant histories of loss report that ending well with their therapist can provide a corrective emotional experience of dealing with loss and endings, which in itself is quite therapeutic.

As a therapist, I enjoy the last stage of the counseling process with my clients, even though it is bittersweet. Together, we celebrate and affirm the changes made and ensure that the new ways of thinking, feeling, and behaving are generalized outside the therapy office to the client's life. We envision new possibilities that did not seem reachable before. We anticipate future challenges and rehearse how they can be surmounted. When I have done my job well in this last phase, clients end their counseling journey with a stronger sense of self-compassion, confidence, and hope that they can navigate life's challenges in the future. Finishing the counseling journey well is essential to ensuring a successful therapy outcome. How do we finish well? I have found that there are five essential tasks to attend to during the end stage of therapy: looking back, looking out, looking in, looking ahead, and looking between.

Looking back. It is often surprising for clients to look back on where they were when they started counseling and realize just how far they have come. The last phase of therapy includes reviewing the initial goals for therapy and affirming the changes that have occurred, which may include growth in areas the client did not envision. This review can consist

---

[3]Joshua K. Swift and Roger P. Greenberg, *Premature Termination in Psychotherapy: Strategies for Engaging Clients and Improving Outcomes* (Washington, DC: American Psychological Association, 2015).

of revisiting journal entries, poetry, artwork, or other modes of self-expression for the client during the therapy journey. If expressive therapies such as art and creative writing have been a part of your work in therapy, you might find that these creative avenues are helpful ways to express the complexity of feelings that often arise at the end of the counseling journey.

Recently, with a client, we reviewed her scores on a symptom checklist, comparing anxiety symptoms at the beginning of counseling (in the severe range) to now (nonclinical range), to her great encouragement. It was a joy to celebrate together and envision what a new normal of living without debilitating anxiety could look like as she began to consider activities and goals that did not seem possible before therapy.

Looking back also includes a reflective review of the counseling experience. I ask clients, "What was the most helpful and important part of our work together? What were the least helpful experiences?" I find this allows for an important review and evaluation of the experience and an opportunity to recognize key moments in therapy that were helpful or difficult. This also provides the opportunity to address any unfinished business the client may have about their experience in treatment. For example, one of my clients recalled that she felt she benefited greatly from the experiential interventions in sessions where we focused on deepening her emotional awareness but did not gain much from homework exercises. She hoped she did not disappoint me with her lack of follow-through on my suggestions for between-session work. I assured her I was not disappointed and that I respected and understood her need to confine the therapeutic work to our scheduled sessions.

As the therapist, I will also share my reflections on the work together as we look back, focusing specifically on key moments where I was inspired by my client's courageous work and learned important lessons from them. It is important to me that my clients know that I, too, am positively affected by the hours we spend together in counseling.

Looking out. An important task of the last stage of therapy is ensuring that the client's new ways of thinking, feeling, and behaving benefit situations outside the therapy office. This application of new knowledge and skills in the client's day-to-day life has likely been ongoing throughout therapy. Still, it is essential in the last stage of treatment to ensure that this generalization has happened. For example, my client Theresa has become much more open, honest, and assertive about her needs and feelings with me in the therapy office. But is she able to do this with family and coworkers? In the last stage of therapy, we ensure that the gains are also applied to the client's day-to-day functioning. Your therapist may suggest a variety of activities that help you with this looking-out process that include role-playing challenging situations or even bringing in significant others for critical conversations to support the changes you have made.

Looking inward. One aspect of affirming client growth and development involves exploring the new, internalized understanding of themselves that has emerged from the counseling experience. What new areas of strength and resilience are evident for you now? Where are the vulnerabilities or triggers that you need to be aware of going forward? A beneficial outcome of therapy for most clients is a greater acceptance and compassion for their human struggles, in contrast to the shame and self-criticism that they have carried before treatment. In the last stage of counseling, you have the opportunity to consider how this more profound and more accurate view of yourself can translate into new possibilities for the future.

Looking ahead. This important part of the last phase of the counseling journey involves anticipating future challenges and developing a plan of action for addressing them. For some clients, this will include relapse-prevention planning, where we anticipate triggers for relapsing into old ways of thinking and acting and envision alternative strategies.

Looking forward, clients can also identify the support needed for their continued growth and development. In place of therapy, for example, they may choose to attend a support group to continue their journey with others who share similar struggles. For some clients, engaging in volunteer work to pass the lessons they have learned on to others is the next step in their growth. In looking to the future with hope, you can begin to envision new opportunities available to you that were not considered before.

Looking between. Perhaps the most challenging and bittersweet task in ending well is looking between and bringing closure to the therapeutic relationship. I have affirmed throughout this book the importance of the therapy relationship as a foundation for growth and change in the counseling process. Saying goodbye well honors the depth and value of the client-therapist relationship and says, "It is hard to say goodbye because you matter to me." Bringing resolution to the therapeutic relationship can provide us with a model of how we can finish well in other relationships. How do we bring closure to this important relationship and say goodbye?

First, we express appreciation and gratitude for our good work together. I take this opportunity to affirm my client's strengths and my hopes for their future. I express to them how much our work together has meant to me and what I have learned from them. I make sure to remind them that the door is always open if they need to return to therapy.

Second, we make sure to clear up any unfinished business between us. We may remember together the ruptures and repairs in the therapeutic relationship. I will check to see whether there are any lingering concerns, questions, or issues that need to be expressed.

When these important tasks are completed, nothing is left to do but celebrate. I love a good celebration, and marking the conclusion of the hard work of counseling with my clients is something I relish. Over the years, celebration sessions have included something as simple as expressions of mutual appreciation, enjoying a special food or beverage together, or sharing a prayer. One client and I developed a short liturgy for the completion of his counseling, expressing gratitude to God for his suffering redeemed. I have had child clients who insisted on party hats and noisemakers for their final session. What could be better to celebrate than improved mental health?

Looking up. For clients of faith, we can add a sixth task to ending well in therapy: expressing gratitude to God for the healing journey. We humbly acknowledge our dependence on God's providence and provision throughout the counseling experience and seek his guidance and wisdom for the future. I often find that clients will still come to mind long after we have had our last therapy session, and when this occurs, I see it as a prompt from God to pray for their continued well-being.

Anticipating Potential Challenges and Maintaining the Gains Made in Therapy

I briefly touched on this topic as an important part of *looking forward* near the end of the counseling journey. In the last stage of therapy, the client and therapist need to work together to anticipate potential future challenges so the hard-earned gains made in treatment can be maintained. You may be familiar with the principle of homeostasis, which posits that most organisms, including human systems, seek to maintain consistency and equilibrium. If we introduce change to the system, it upsets the equilibrium (even if the constant state is unhealthy), and the system exerts internal pressure to return to the usual way of functioning.

You will likely experience subtle internal and external pressure to return to your old ways of functioning, as your new ways of thinking and acting may disrupt the balance of the groups you are a part of. Maintaining the gains made in therapy involves using the last stage of therapy to predict and prepare for the response of your environment to the changes you have made.

I worked for several years as the director of an inpatient adolescent unit. We would work hard with patients to address their problem behaviors and unhealthy (and often self-destructive) coping. But then, inevitably, we would send them home to their family system, and they would fall back into old behavior patterns. We found we had to help the family together find a new way of functioning to support the changes of their teenager. Maybe the teen's acting-out behavior had taken the focus of the marital discord between husband and wife and forced them to form a parenting partnership. Without intervention, there would be unconscious pressure on the teen to resume their behavior to serve the needed function for the family.

Another related task in the last stage of therapy involves relapse prevention. I will often predict to clients that they may have times when they find themselves falling back on old patterns and habits, but brief relapses are to be expected and signal to us that we need to strengthen our support or find better ways to cope with certain triggers. Addiction specialists offer a number of helpful ways to prevent relapses, including the following:[4]

- Relapse is often a gradual process, and it is important to be able to recognize the early signs so we can take action.

- Recovery from addictions and problem behaviors is a lifelong process, and no matter how far along we are, there are risks of relapse at every stage.

- Acquiring and practicing good coping skills and stress management skills is important for preventing relapse.

- Be honest if you are struggling and seek help.

If you find yourself unable to get back on your feet after a relapse, do not despair. It is time to reconnect with your therapist for help getting back on track.

HOW DO I KNOW WHETHER I NEED TO RETURN TO THERAPY?

Many clients find it helpful to periodically return to therapy during periods of crisis or for help and support in maintaining the gains made in treatment. As discussed above, it is common for clients to experience brief periods of relapse or fall back into old habits after the end of therapy. Most often, clients are able to get themselves back on track using the self-knowledge and skills learned in therapy.

However, if symptoms and problems persist beyond a few weeks, scheduling a follow-up session with your therapist may be helpful. Some specific indicators that a return to therapy is needed include the following:

- persistent thoughts of harming self or others
- symptoms are interfering with day-to-day functioning (school, work, family life)
- loss, transition, or changes that are difficult to navigate alone

---

[4] Steven M. Melemis, "Relapse Prevention and the Five Rules of Recovery," *The Yale Journal of Biology and Medicine* 88, no. 3 (2015): 325-32, https://pubmed.ncbi.nlm.nih.gov /26339217/.

- recognition of falling back into old patterns with difficulty finding a way out
- a new set of symptoms emerges that parallel previous difficulties (i.e., you use therapy to successfully quit smoking but find yourself falling into compulsive overeating habits)
- a desire for a check-in session to ensure that the gains made in therapy are maintained and sustained

Often, people find it helpful to return to therapy at different points in their lives to engage in a new or deeper exploration of issues. While there can be benefits to returning to a trusted therapist who knows your history, it is also perfectly acceptable to find a new therapist who may have a different expertise or approach to counseling.

Therapeutic Boundaries After the Completion of Therapy

Inevitably, as we bring closure to the therapy relationship, questions arise about keeping in touch following the end of therapy. Clients may inquire about meeting socially, connecting through social media, or exchanging text messages in the future.

Because of the unique nature of the therapeutic relationship, it is not advisable or ethical for clients and counselors to transition to a social relationship after therapy concludes. I will tell clients that while I welcome their future communications and updates, I am responsible for safeguarding their investment of time and money in the therapy process by maintaining therapeutic boundaries even after therapy is finished. Clients likely have many options for friendships in their lifetime but only a few therapists, and I can best care for them by maintaining my professional role in case they need to return to therapy sometime in the future.

I firmly believe that psychotherapy is not something we ever graduate from. Rather, it is most helpful to think of therapy as an available source of support and growth that we can come back to at different points of our lives when we are stuck, sick, or need a place to process (remember the value of liminal space?). This is a compelling reason for your therapist not to engage in a social relationship or friendship with you posttherapy. If you do return for therapy, even if just for a few sessions, you will most likely find it is relatively easy to reconnect with your therapist and pick up right where you left off in your process of growth and development.

Faith Perspectives: Finding Meaning in the Struggle

The end stage of the counseling journey provides a rich opportunity for clients to reflect on their experiences of adversity and suffering and potentially discover that these difficult experiences indeed have meaning. Perhaps a sense of gratitude emerges for you for the changes you have been able to make in response to adverse circumstances. Or you may feel a greater sense of purpose for your life has developed from the healing journey. Sometimes the meaning may be a renewed sense of personal and spiritual resiliency from surviving an excruciatingly difficult situation through the experience of God's faithfulness in the midst of suffering.

Psychologists use the term *posttraumatic growth* to describe the phenomena of positive growth and changes following experiences of adversity.[5] Experiences of suffering often trigger the reevaluation of our cherished beliefs about ourselves and the world. Through the counseling journey, clients explore the hard questions as they seek to make sense of their adverse experiences and find meaning and purpose for their lives. In the last stage of therapy, clients are often able to see how their suffering has been transformative as they emerge from the counseling journey with greater resilience and hope, improved relationships, or a renewed sense of calling and vocation.

We can look at the Old Testament narrative of Joseph in Genesis as evidence of God's redemptive work. Sold into slavery by his brothers, Joseph suffered betrayal, imprisonment, and humiliation only to eventually rise to the ranks of influence with the king. His brothers, however, faced famine in their own lands and were sent to beg the king for mercy, only to realize the king's representative was none other than their younger

---

[5]Richard Tedeshi and Lawrence G. Calhoun, *Posttraumatic Growth: Conceptual Foundation and Empirical Evidence* (Philadelphia: Lawrence Erlbaum Associates, 2004).

brother, whom they had left for dead. In a decisive moment of redemption, Joseph gifts them the needed grain and says, "You intended to harm me, but God intended it for good to accomplish what is now being done, the saving of many lives" (Genesis 50:20).

Redemption of suffering is God's specialty, a beautiful mystery that happens again and again as we are formed in Christ's likeness. For God's people, we are familiar with the transformative journey with God of fall and redemption, sin and grace, confession and forgiveness. We see these themes in the grand narrative of Scripture and in our own lives. As therapists, we see these redemptive themes play out in tangible ways in the therapy office as clients evidence faith, hope, and love following experiences of great adversity. When we cannot see purpose in our own suffering, we can borrow hope from the many examples we see in history and Scripture of God's redemptive actions with his people.

Action Step: Giving Back

For some clients, making meaning from their suffering involves a new sense of purpose or calling to use their knowledge and experience to help others who are suffering in similar ways. I think of the client I worked with whose healing journey from trauma led him to use his story to speak to students about risk and prevention strategies around sexual assault, or the couple who struggled through a process of forgiveness and reconciliation in their marriage who now provide mentoring for other couples in similar circumstances. We all know inspiring examples of people who bring tremendous credibility and experience in helping others as part of their continued healing journey.

Psychologist and researcher Judith Herman has spent her career learning from people who have experienced interpersonal trauma, including abuse, neglect, and intimate partner violence. She writes:

> Most survivors seek the resolution of their traumatic experience within the confines of their personal lives. But a significant minority, as a result of the trauma, feel called upon to engage in a wider world. These survivors recognize a political or religious

dimension in their misfortune, and discover that they can transform the meaning of their personal tragedy by making it the basis for social action. While there is no way to compensate for an atrocity, there is a way to transcend it, by making it a gift to others. The trauma is redeemed only when it becomes the source of a survivor mission.[6]

This quote brings to mind respected colleagues who recognize their own mental health journeys as the impetus for the counseling practices they have built to help clients through difficulties similar to what they themselves have experienced. Their thriving practices today are a beautiful testimony to God's redemption of suffering, which is at the heart of their desire to provide others with a pathway to healing.

Over the years, it has been a sacred honor to see many clients find a true passion and calling that comes out of their own experiences of suffering and healing. Considering potential opportunities for the redemption of suffering can be part of this last stage of the counseling process for you, providing meaning, purpose, and passion for the journey onward.

Summing Up

We have explored in this chapter the significant growth opportunities available during the last stage of the counseling journey as you have the opportunity to celebrate the gains you have made, carry forward changes and new insights, and perhaps recognize the transformative impact of your suffering through a new sense of meaning and purpose. While it is bittersweet to bring the therapy relationship to a close, ending well can provide a corrective experience for dealing authentically and meaningfully with life's experiences of loss. Your preparation work during the last phase of therapy will give you confidence to navigate future challenges and ensure that you will continue to experience the benefits of therapy long after your counseling journey has come to a close. As you

[6]Judith L. Herman, "Recovery from Psychological Trauma," *Psychiatry and Clinical Neurosciences* 52 (1998): S98-S103, https://onlinelibrary.wiley.com/doi/10.1046/j.1440-1819.1998.0520s5S145.x.

finish the counseling journey, you can go forward into the future with hope and confidence, resting assured that the therapy office door is always open to you if you get stuck or sidetracked along the way.

Roles Recap: Ending Well

THERAPIST ROLES	CLIENT ROLES
Regularly assess the client's progress toward therapy goals	Self-monitor symptoms and report your progress to your therapist
Initiate collaborative conversations with clients about their readiness to end therapy	Engage in collaborative conversations about your readiness to end therapy
Encourage clients to review and reflect on their therapy experience	Reflect on the therapy experience, both benefits and challenges
Recommend activities to generalize the gains made in therapy to the client's daily life	Apply the gains made in therapy to your daily life
Explore potential future challenges and foster relapse prevention	Identify areas of needed support for continued growth and development
Foster posttraumatic growth through identifying resilience and encouraging meaning-making	Reflect on the meaning and purpose of adverse experiences in your life
Maintain boundaries posttherapy and invite clients to return as needed	Celebrate changes and engage in life!

Against an Infinite Horizon

I love the experience of looking out over a body of water that appears to stretch endlessly to a horizon, where it is indeterminate where the water ends and the sky begins. For me, this view evokes such a sense of eternity and mystery. Similarly, I find much meaning in adopting an eternal perspective on the counseling journey as one brief human encounter against an infinite horizon of eternal life with God and his people. "To have faith is to see everything against an infinite horizon," writes Father Ron Rolheiser.[1] By faith, I trust that the sacred relationships I have with my clients will continue beyond the end of counseling, even the end of this life, with eternal significance.

Clients often find that they have internalized (hopefully the best) aspects of their therapist that they carry forward and can draw from as needed during their continued journey toward human flourishing. I have clients tell me how they can hear my voice in their heads when they get in a jam, and I hope and pray that my internalized words are ones of encouragement, caring, and empowerment. An essential part of the process of grief and loss is our ability to carry the thoughts and memories of significant others with us, even when they are no longer present in our day-to-day lives. The truth is that we, too, as therapists, carry our clients with us long after termination. Your stories, your struggles, and your courage and resilience in the face of suffering are some of the many ways you also become a part of us.

I can think of no better way to finish *The Client's Guide to Therapy* than to let you know that the counseling journey is mutually transformative for both the client and the therapist. You need to know that as therapists, we, too, are transformed by our work with you as our clients. Accompanying you through the wilderness is a sacred calling, and we

---

[1]Ronald Rolheiser, *Against an Infinite Horizon: The Finger of God in Our Everyday Lives* (New York: Crossroad, 2002), 9.

are honored to be entrusted with your innermost thoughts and feelings. Our time with you changes us as we have a front-row seat to your healing and transformation. We are inspired by your courage, deeply moved by your suffering, and experience great joy in your hard-won progress. We are also challenged by your example to continue in our own psychological and spiritual journeys in more faithful and loving ways. As your therapists, we owe you a debt of gratitude for the people we are today.

Thank you for allowing me to be a part of your journey through the pages of *The Client's Guide to Therapy.* I hope I have imparted my absolute confidence that, truly, the meaningful and transformative counseling journey is yours for the taking. You have already accomplished a significant step by reading this book and equipping yourself with the knowledge and skills you need for a successful counseling experience— great job! Now, I invite you to consider your next step prayerfully. Have you found a counselor yet? If not, do not delay any longer. Share your intentions to see a therapist with a family member or friend. Reread the action steps in chapter two and be persistent in finding a therapist to begin this journey with. Remember all the compelling reasons to see a therapist as described in chapter one and take the next step toward improving your mental health, quality of life, spiritual vitality, and resilience. If you are already in counseling, I hope you have highlighted and marked up sections of this book to discuss with your therapist that can provide trail markers and guideposts to help you navigate the therapy process. You can do this!

If, after reading this book, you recognize that you are not yet ready or able to pursue counseling, I hope that the action steps and self-assessment questions provide opportunities to reflect on your own spiritual and mental health. You may find benefit in discussing your questions and insights with a trusted mentor, small group, or pastor. Healing occurs in the context of relationships, including all kinds of significant others in addition to the therapy relationship.

Finally, as a fellow traveler, I offer you this prayer, which expresses my confidence and hope for you as you follow our ultimate trustworthy and true Guide:

The LORD will guide you always;
> he will satisfy your needs in a sun-scorched land
> and will strengthen your frame.
You will be like a well-watered garden,
> like a spring whose waters never fail. (Isaiah 58:11)

General Index